D1454613

Cornelius Stetter

The Secret Medicine of the Pharaohs

Ancient Egyptian Healing

edition q

Chicago · Berlin · Moscow · Tokyo

Title of the original German edition: Denn alles steht seit Ewigkeit geschrieben — Die geheime Medizin der Pharaonen. Quintessence Publishing Co., Munich 1990.

Library of Congress
Cataloging-in-Publication Data
Stetter, Cornelius.
[Denn alles steht seit Ewigkeit geschrieben. English]
The secret medicine of the pharaohs : ancient Egyptian medicine /
Cornelius Stetter.
p.   cm.
Includes bibliographical references.
ISBN 0-86715-265-6
1. Medicine, Egyptian. 2. History of Medicine, Ancient--Egypt. I. Title.
[DNLM: WZ 70 HE3 S8d 1993a]
R 137. S7413 1993
610'.932—dc20
DNLM/DLC
for Library of Congress   92-48470
                                       CIP

© 1993 by Edition Q, a Division of Quintessence Publishing Co, Inc, Carol Stream, Illinois.

Lithography: Toppan Printing Co. (S) Pte., Ltd., Singapore, and JuP Industrie- und Presseklischee, Berlin
Typesetting: av-satz, Berlin
Printing, and Binding: Bosch-Druck, Landshut/Ergolding

Contents

7   **Introduction**
The Land and Its People Over
5,000 Years

21   **Prologue**
How the Hieroglyphs Were
Rediscovered

25   **The Secrets of the Papyri**

45   **How an Illness Develops**

51   **May the Heart be Happy**
Medical Life in Egypt

65   **Imhotep**
The Doctor Who Became a God

69   **Disease and Deformity**
Obesity, Hunchbacks, and Dwarfs

81   **Travels With Hatshepsut**

85   **Love, Lust, and Birth**

91   **Practical Therapeutics**
"First the teeth, then the eyes"

101   **Magical-Religious Treatments**

107   **Remedies**
From the Electric Ray to the Poppy

123   **Body Maintenance and Care**
Hygiene and Circumcision

Contents

135   **Spiritual and Divine Order**

141   **The Book of the Dead**

147   **The Trip to the Other Side**

169   **Epilogue**

173   **Glossary**

179   **References**

Introduction

The Land and Its People Over 5,000 Years

The history of medicine in ancient Egypt would not be complete without at least a short description of the land in which, several thousand years ago, so many uncommon things took place. How was it possible that 5,000 years ago, in the endless, desolate Sahara desert, such an extraordinary culture could develop? Many puzzles of this mysterious land have a common key: the Nile.

Egypt is a child of the Nile. Ancient Egyptians did not know (or did not want to know) where the river came from; they thought that it came from the sky. The "White Nile" rises in the lakes of equatorial Africa more than 6,500 kilometers from the Nile's estuary. After half of its course is run, it unites with the "Blue Nile," a rapid mountainous river rising in the Ethiopian highlands. Then, 320 kilometers further, the longest river on earth joins its last tributary: the Atbara. With further windings, it finds its way over five falls (or cataracts), the farthest north of which is in the region of Aswan, the Syene of antiquity. Here the Nile valley suddenly becomes an emerald green of vegetation stripes in the middle of the brutal yellow desert, which each day before sunset turn to violet. One thousand three hundred kilometers further, the Nile fans to a delta. Annually, between July and October (the snow-melting and rainy seasons in central Africa), the Nile increases to a rapid stream which brings rich soil from middle Africa to Egypt. The flooding water leaves the fertile mud behind, the basis for Egypt's prosperity—when the inundation does not occur—famine. (Today, such Nile mud is missing. Between 1959 and 1970, the President of Egypt, Gamal Abdel Nasser, introduced the prestigious "Sadd al-Ali," the construction of a 3.8-kilometer-long and 111-meter-high Aswan dam behind which is the 500-kilometer-long Lake Nasser. The fertile Nile mud now collects on the dam wall, which regularly results in clogging of almost all the turbines. Experts maintain that in the not-too-distant future the lake will overflow because the mud will have reached the height of the wall.)

In early Egyptian history, the land was divided into forty-two districts: twenty along the valley and twenty-two in the delta. In time, various clans united and formed the two kingdoms of Upper and Lower Egypt. The kings from Upper Egypt took as their symbol a white crown with a vulture. The kings of Lower Egypt used a red crown and their totem animal was the cobra. Later, when the two kingdoms united, the pharaoh used the so-called double crown. The union is also represented in many pictures with plants: interwoven are lotus flowers and papyrus, which are typical plants of Upper and Lower Egypt.

In addition to the Nile val-ley and the delta, there was a third, larger and inhabited region: the Faiyum, a lake oasis south of Memphis. Today, it still receives influx through Bahr Jusuf, a branching Nile arm north of Asyut which flows westward and ends in Karun Lake (Birket Qarun) in the Moëris Lake of ancient times. The word is of old Egyptian origin and means more or less "big lake." Since the early time of Christianity, the Egyptians called it Pa-jom (the sea), and this name was transformed into today's "Faiyum." The lake is forty-five meters below sea level and is about forty kilometers long. In ancient days, it was six times larger and teemed with crocodiles. Sobek, the crocodile god, was therefore the male deity of this region. By the construction of powerful locks, it was possible to force the lake into a smaller area and to obtain fruitful land, which could bring two harvests a year. Pharaoh Senwosret II started these enormous cultivation efforts and Amenemhet III completed them. He ordered the construction of a pyramid with a "lake view," which today has almost completely disappeared. The death temple—300 x 240 meters in size—in antiquity was considered a famous labyrinth. Strabo[1] reported that in 25 BC it was not possible for a foreigner to go through the courts and ways without a guide. According to a Greek legend, Daedalus constructed a labyrinth in the palace at Knosos on Crete in which the mon-

---

[1] Greek geographer, 63 BC – ? AD 24.

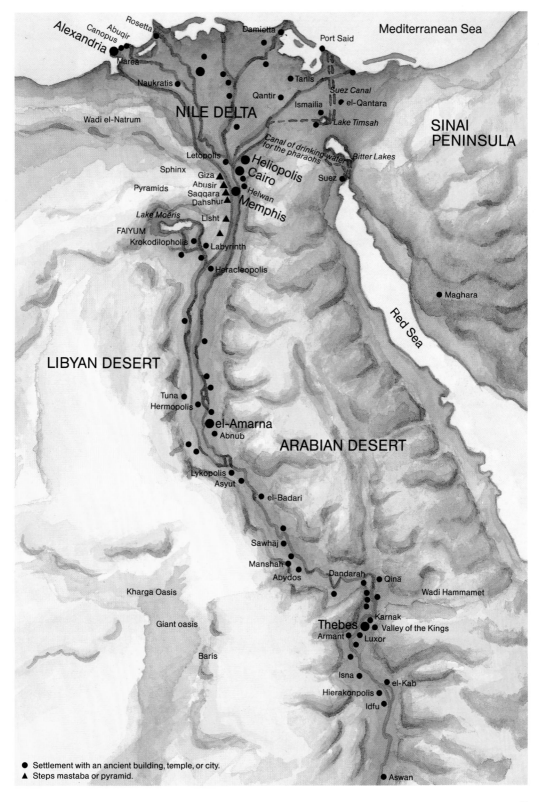

Alexandria
Abuqir
Canopus
Rosetta
Damietta
Port Said
Mediterranean Sea
Marea
Tanis
Suez Canal
Naukratis
Qantir
Ismailia
el-Qantara
NILE DELTA
Lake Timsah
SINAI
PENINSULA
Wadi el-Natrum
Canal of drinking water
for the pharaohs
Bitter Lakes
Letopolis
Heliopolis
Sphinx
Cairo
Giza ▲
Suez
Pyramids
Abusir ▲
Saqqara ▲
Helwan
Dahshur ▲
Memphis
Lake Moëris
Lisht ▲
▲
FAIYUM
Krokodilopolis
Labyrinth
Heracleopolis
Maghara
LIBYAN DESERT
Red Sea
Tuna
Hermopolis
el-Amarna
Abnub
ARABIAN DESERT
Lykopolis
Asyut
el-Badari
Sawhāj
Kharga Oasis
Manshah
Abydos
Dandarah
Qinā
Wadi Hammamet
Giant oasis
Thebes
Karnak
Valley of the Kings
Armant
Luxor
Baris
Isna
el-Kab
Hierakonpolis
Idfu

● Settlement with an ancient building, temple, or city.
▲ Steps mastaba or pyramid.

Aswan

9

Period	Time*	Dynasty	Most important pharaohs
Prehistory and early dynastic period	5000–2686 BC		
Old Kingdom	2686–2613	III	Djoser; Huni
	2613–2494	IV	Snofru; Cheops; Khephren; Mycerinus
	2494–2345	V	Sahure; Neuserre; Wenis
	2345–2181	VI	Pepy I; Pepy II
First Intermediate Period	2134–2040		Numerous kings until the XIth Dynasty in Memphis, Heracleopolis, and Thebes: Khety; Merykare; Inyotef; Mentuhotpe
Middle Kingdom	2040–1991	XI	Mentuhotpe
	1991–1786	XII	Amenemhet I to IV; Senwosret I–III
	until 1640	XIII	
		XIV	About 100 different kings
Second Intermediate Period	until 1550	XV	
		XVI	Numerous kings
		XVII	
New Kingdom	1550–1070	XVIII	Amenophis I–III; Akhenaten; Aya; Tuthmosis I–III; Haremhab; Smenkhkare (Nefertiti?); Hatshepsut; Tutankhamun
		XIX	Sethos I, II; Ramses I, II; Merneptah
		XX	Ramses III–XI

nd Their Rulers

Period	Time	Dynasty	Most important pharaohs
Third Intermediate Period	1070–712	XXI–XXV	About 25 kings. (In the XXIIIrd Dynasty there were more simultaneous king's courts in Thebes, Hermopolis, Tanis, Heracleopolis, Leontopolis)
Late Period	712–332	XXVI XXVII XXVIII– XXX XXXI	Psammetichus I to III Darius; Xerxes Amyrtaios until Nectanebo II Second Persian period. Darius III. In this time the Nubian King Khababash ruled Egypt for a short time; Alexander the Great
Greco-Roman Period	332 BC– AD 395		Ptolemaic Dynasty (Ptolemy I–XV; Cleopatra); Roman emperors after 30 BC: Augustus; Tiberius; Caligula; Claudius; Nero ...

* Despite varied research, the dates, at least in the Old and Middle Kingdoms are not defined. We must be content with approximations. After the New Kingdom, the documents became more precise.

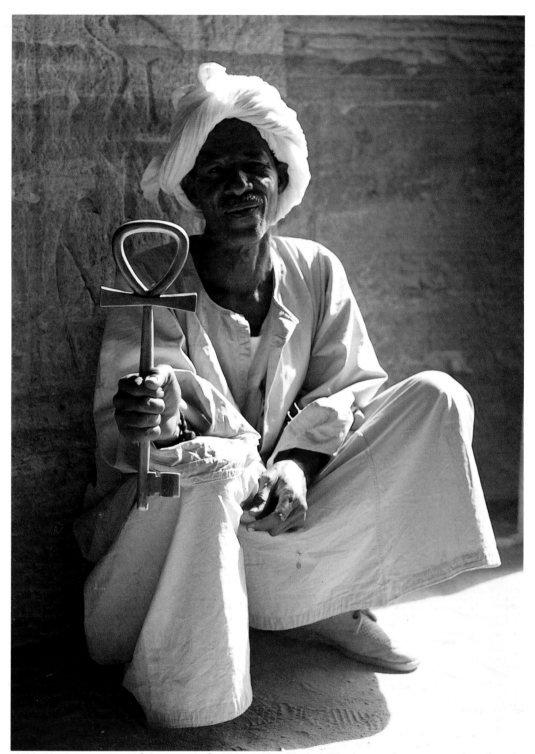

Abdul is the guardian of the temple facility at Abu Simbel. The key to the entrance door has the "ankh" sign, the symbol of life force.

ster "Minotaurus," a creature half man, half steer, lived. Diodor from Sicily[2] wrote that this Greek labyrinth was only a small copy of the Egyptian labyrinth. For Herodotus[3] there was even more—namely 1,500 subterranean rooms with chambers for twelve pharaohs. To date, they have not been found during the excavations. The labyrinth awaits a modern Schliemann.[4]

"Although the labyrinth is a real miracle the closely located Moëris lake is a bigger one," wrote Herodotus, "its circumference is 3,600 Stadium, which is the length of the whole coast of Egypt." Linant Pascha found 1,842 marks in the old dams. Therefore, the old lake must have had a surface of 157 square kilometers—an unimaginable water system!

Herodotus must have seen the lake in its original size, because it filled with sand in Roman times when no pharaoh was concerned with the water reservoir; the Egyptian kingdom was "closed." Periods of drought and sand-filling left the Moëris lake smaller and smaller. (As an example of how fast these occurrences take place in these areas, when Lake Nasser lost the affluence of the Ethiopian part due to drought in 1968, the water level of the 5,000-kilometer lake lowered by thirty-five meters!)

[2] Diodorus Siculus, Greek historian, first century BC.
[3] Greek historian, fifth century BC.
[4] Heinrich Schliemann (1822–1890), German archaeologist.

A region very similar to the Faiyum was the Wadi el-Natrum, an oasis at the Delta, south of Alexandria. "Natrum" refers to the salt lakes located there in which sodium bicarbonate, important for mummification, was obtained.

The Nile had other wide-reaching effects on Egyptian society. The calendar year began when the flood arrived. The year was composed of three time periods of four months each: the time of flooding, the month of planting and growing, and the time of harvest. The month had thirty days, the year had 360 days. To these, five extra days were added in which the birthdays of the five main deities were celebrated. Soon the Egyptians discovered that the year did not have 365 days but $365\frac{1}{4}$, but the peasants followed a sun calendar.

The classic source for Egyptian history is the pharaoh list, which was recorded in the third century BC by Manetho. Manetho was a priest in Heliopolis and completed this work for Ptolemy II. The original (Greek) manuscript did not survive, so we must base our knowledge on the transcripts of the early historians Flavius Josephus, Sextus Julius Africanus, or Eusebius of Ceasarea. Manetho starts his list of kings with a man he calls Menes and with the union of Upper and Lower Egypt. The succeeding ruler-dynasties are then collected into historical periods: the Old Kingdom, Middle Kingdom, and New Kingdom. In the "intermediate periods" there are documentations, of breaks in the uniform course of Egyptian history (these touch in part on invasions of foreign people).

The residence of the kings and the central point of administration was at Memphis and occurred after the consolidation of the Upper and Lower Kingdoms. Close by was the burial area in Saqqara, which by the end of the pharaoh reigns had become a major city for dead kings, important persons, and millions of mummified, sacred animals.

Pharaohs, court employees, the first scribes, priests, and physicians of these early centuries of the first dynasties were of an impressive genius. They "invented" the calendar, paper, and writing, obtained remarkable results in geometry, devised impressive water systems, and were not to be surpassed in their skill of storage and logistics. In the first dynasty—more than 5,000 years ago—the Egyptians had a decimal system and could calculate the surface of a triangle, a square, a trapezoid, or even a circle. In the latter case, they constructed a square of eight-ninths of the diameter which gave a value to the number Pi of 3.1605. Only in the year AD 1596 did the circular number, which the analysts must have known for the construction of the pyramids, enter our mathematics. At that time, the Dutch professor Ludolph van Ceulen calculated it as 3.14159265358979323846.

Also, the knowledge of physics in the early dynasties of ancient Egypt must have been rather advanced. We assume today that Benjamin Franklin invented the lightning rod about 200 years ago. However, in the fifteenth century BC, the temples were constructed in such a manner that entrance took place through the central door (the so-called Pylon) which was flanked by two high fortress-like turrets. Each of these turrets contained two gutters, each of which held a "mast-tree." These mast-trees were very tall; in the temple of Edfu, they were 100 feet high (about thirty meters). An inscription of the Ptolemy was found there. It read, "This is the height of the Pylon construction of the god of Edfu, at the main site of the lightning horn; mast-trees are found parallel here, to cut the tempest in the sky." And also by the rules of conductivity of electricity, it seems the Egyptians knew that metal is a good conductor and copper a better one. Also, the Ptolemy reported, "these mast-trees are covered with copper to better fulfill their function."

The discovery of writing (and of writing material, which was so much more practical than the totem poles of the Babylonians) influenced the social structure considerably. Writing was important for the administration of the land, and men who were able to read and write, or able to record appropriately, became important persons in the kingdom. To that point, society was made up of two classes: on one side was the nobility with regional princes, the governors, officials, and warriors; on the other side were the peasants and manual workers. With the advent of writing, a new class developed: people knowledgeable in writing who could become high officers or physicians.

The Old Kingdom reached its high point at the time of the construction of the great pyramids of Snofru, Khufu (Cheops), Khephren, and Menkaure (Mycerinus) during the Fourth Dynasty. Previously, King Djoser had set an example with the oldest pyramid of the world, in Saqqara. Nothing so powerful had been built by men before that time, and this is also amazing in Egyptian history. Suddenly, 5,000 years ago, humankind made a major step forward. Without preparation, advanced civilization developed with breathtaking technical highpoints. A civilization was able to move in all directions. Certainly, the pyramid construction was a milestone in the history of humankind, since, for the first time, a form of technology of major breadth was utilized and problems that resulted from this were resolved.

The workforce formed a united country, where one could not forget that it had a common religion. The almost unimaginable work involved in pyramid construction would not have been possible with forced labor. The oldest pyramid of Saqqara resulted from the work of a genial vizier of Lower Egypt, the first after the king of Upper Egypt, head of the courts, owner of the hereditary nobility, high priest of Heliopolis, constructor, sculptor, and highest "vase creator": Imhotep—physician, and known by the Greeks later as the god of cures, Asklepios.

Without doubt, the pyramid of the Pharaoh Khufu (Cheops)— one of the seven marvels of the world—is not only the biggest, but also the one constructed with greatest care. With mathematical precision, the four sides are directed in the four compass directions. The construction covers an area of 230 meters as a side, and the mass of the pyramid is made of about 6.5 million tons of limestone. In a length of 230 meters there is only a sixteen-millimeter deviation from the right angle! (One should think of a normal room ceiling, which in an average of five meters, has a height difference of two centimeters.) The pyramid had a height of 146.6 meters (now 137 meters) and a sloping angle of fifty-two degrees. That is, it has the unique geometrical property that its height is in the same relation to its circumference as the radius of a circle is to the circumference $(1:2)$. The pyramid was measured exactly, and one notices that the relationship numbers were kept at the precision of one one-thousandth. Since this cannot be an accident, the wildest speculations have taken place. Even today the construction of the pyramid would cause great technical and organizational problems. The project was finished in twenty-three years. This means that each year about 100,000 stone blocks, with an average weight of two and a half tons (there are some which weigh forty tons), had to be cut, trimmed, transported by the

Nile from the quarries to Giza, then transported for kilometers through the desert, and finally used in the construction—about 285 blocks each day! With a work day of twelve hours, this means that each two and a half minutes, a square stone weighing a ton was set in place. No one has been able to definitely determine or explain how this took place. There are no drawings.

With the growth of the construction, the stone blocks had to be transported higher and higher, and the work surface became smaller and smaller, so that at the end cartage animals could no longer be used. Machines with wheels did not exist so the stones had to be transported by ramps and sledges.

The maintenance of the workers must also have been an immense problem if we consider only the 100,000 employed as reported by Herodotus (other sources speak of about 280,000). Erik von Däniken has a humorous calculation; since the Egyptians enjoyed radishes and onions, and the foods were part of the daily ration (there was even a radish strike), he concluded: if we consider that one worker consumes only a 100-gram onion a day, then 100,000 workers would eat 10,000 kilos of onions daily, or 300 tons a month. If they worked only half a year on the construction, they had to bring 1,800 tons of onions to the site. Since there were no trucks, the onions had to be transported in sacks on boats and from these with oxen and mules.

Hence, there would be 200 workers busy with the transport alone of 50-kilo sacks and the unloading and distribution. However, the workers did not live on onions alone ....

The original entrance of the pyramid was on its north side, adjusted to the polar star, at a height of 18 meters. At that point, there is a ninety-seven-meter walkway with an inclination downwards of twenty-seven degrees into the earth into a tomb chamber. Another thirty-eight-meter, very low walkway leads to the inside from the floor space upwards. It then continues horizontally and goes higher so that people may walk upright. This walk ends in a room, precisely under the tip, which is twenty meters above ground level. Another walkway ends blindly, and the incomplete floor makes us assume that this plan had been discontinued. It goes up forty-two meters and is called "the big gallery" because of its height of more than eight meters.

The gallery leads to the tomb chamber, which is covered with black granite and is directly under the tip of the pyramid. The sarcophagus was empty at its discovery and the cover had disappeared. It is believed that during the time of the Old Kingdom, the workers entered the pyramid.

In order to picture the enormous size of the pyramid, imagine this comparison: there is space inside the pyramid for the Church of St Peter in Rome, the cathedrals of

Milan and Florence, the London Cathedral of St Paul, and Westminster-Abbey—the five largest churches in the world.

During the centuries after the major pharaohs of the Old Kingdom, a change occurred in the concept of godlikeness of the kings. The highest god revered became the sun, "Re," and the pharaoh was considered the "son of Re." The priests and regional princes strove for more personal power and divided the government. The provincial chiefs transformed their offices into hereditary positions and considered their regions as personal properties that they even protected with arms. Later they also demanded the dignity of the royalty. Famines developed and the Old Kingdom declined. The First Intermediate Period occurred, Egypt was divided again, and the sites of government became Heracleopolis and Thebes.

The Middle Kingdom began in the Eleventh Dynasty and, in a united Egypt, construction started again. The rulers of the Twelfth Dynasty brought to the land internal peace by "clipping the wings" of the region princes. In Lower Nubia, a series of large fortresses were constructed. The influence of Egypt extended to the second Nile cataract and put in place a lively commerce and work in the mountain (eg, gold, diorite). The business relationship with the Middle East was intensified, and the swamps of Faiyum were drained and settled. However, what makes this time interval a "classic period" are the intellectual activities. Relevant literary works were created, which later, in the Eighteenth Dynasty, became classics.

The "Adventures of Sinuhe" became a classic work on the adventure of an Egyptian court officer abroad, as did the "Stories of the Shipwrecked," the stories from the "Papyrus Westcar," and even the "Stories of the 1,001 Nights."

The most remarkable pharaoh of these times was Senwosret III, who had at his disposal a large, permanent army. He controlled gold-rich Nubia, secured the commercial routes to Palestine, and changed the velocity of the first cataracts of the Nile with the construction of channels.

Around 1640 BC, a group of foreigners (from the northern part of Mesopotamia) replaced the Thirteenth Dynasty. It was called "Hyksos," according to a Greek account of the Egyptian concept of "Lords of the Foreign Lands." It was not until 1532 BC that Ahmose (1550–1525 BC) was able to throw the Hyksos out completely. He persecuted them for years, all the way to Palestine, even while engaging in battle in the south, in Nubia, at the island of Sai, at the level of the third cataract, and with internal rebellions he had to quell. However, Ahmose succeeded everywhere and left an intact state. His successor, Amenophis I, was the first pharaoh to construct a tomb in the Valley of the Kings.

Two mountain cuts—an eastward one with the majority of the pharaoh tombs, and a westward one with the tomb of Amenophis III and Ejes—form the "Valley of the Kings." In total, there are 62 opened tombs, the last one being the one of Tutankhamun, which was only discovered in this century by the English archaeologist, Howard Carter. (On the morning of November 6, 1922, he sent to his sponsor, the Earl of Carnavon, this telegram: "Finally wonderful discovery made in the valley; fabulous tomb with intact closure; have closed same, till your arrival. Congratulations.")

Tutankhamun's is the smallest of the tombs, all of which are made in the same manner. In the massive rock, there is a passage (in the case of Haremhab's tomb it is 105 meters deep), which descends and is interrupted by several rooms. The passage ends in a tomb chamber, whose walls are luxuriously and artfully painted, usually with illustrations of religious "books" such as the *Book of Gates*, the *Book of Hell*, or the *Litany of Re* (hymns to Re).

We are unable to imagine how expensive the enormous tomb constructions must have been. The treasury of Tutankhamun is the only one that can give us a small idea. The treasures were contained in two miniscule chambers and today cover the whole first floor of the enormous Egyptian Museum in Cairo. Possibly this treasure was not even typical of the magnificence of splendor of the pharaohs.

The necropolis workers, handworkers, and artists lived near the tombs. In a depression behind the mountain in back of Qurnet Murai are the ruins of about seventy houses in which the workers lived, beginning during the reign of Tuthmosis I. The workers were paid in natural products such as fish, meat, corn, salt, wine, and vegetables.

Tuthmosis I, who took over from the Hyksos the chariot, was one of the boldest generals of ancient Egypt. He undertook extensive wars into the south and west and enlarged the region to the Euphrates river. Tuthmosis III subjugated the Mitanni Kingdom in seventeen campaigns. Under his government, Egypt became the center of the world, and Hittites, Babylonians, and Assyrians hurried to send legations to Egypt. Egypt was never stronger or richer than during this time. The wars brought many slaves, thus cheap labor, into the land. From all directions came tributes in the form of gold, jewels, woods, textiles, and drugs, and all went into Egypt's coffers.

Amenophis IV subsequently neglected external politics and created a religious commotion. With the town of Akhetaten (now Tel el-Amarna), he created a new capital. Amenophis IV decreed that instead of the god Amun, the sun Aton was to be observed as the major deity. The "heretic king," called Akhenaten, wanted the union of the gods. He apparently also wanted to restrict the power of the priests. During the

New Kingdom, the priests owned 750,000 acres of land, 500,000 cattle, and 107,000 slaves. They received taxes from 196 cities and received from the pharaoh (these figures refer to Ramses III) 32,000 kilos of gold, 1 million kilos of silver, and 185,000 sacks of corn—annually!

Akhenaten died without leaving heirs. In the short run, he was unable to convince the people of his religion. All remained as it was before, and his statues were destroyed and his name removed. The ensuing Sethos I, Ramses II, and Siptah, all remarkable men who used the double crown, were unable to stop the decline of the New Kingdom.

When the Bronze Age ended, the Egyptian troops faced warriors with iron weapons. The customs deteriorated, people were not cared for efficiently, justice and administration were as corrupt as the priesthood. Tomb thefts took on alarming proportions; no tomb escaped defilement. Mummies were dismembered or their bandages were removed so that jewels could be stolen. Gold was removed from coffins and silver was fused in place. On the twenty-second day of the third month of the winter season, in the sixteenth year of the reign of Ramses IX (1124 BC), the tomb sculptor Amun-penufer made the following statement during a trial: "We found the royal mummy of the sacred king who was armed with this curved saber. Innumerable amulets and jewels were on his chest, and a gold mask was on his face. The royal mummy of this king was totally covered with gold and his coffins were decorated with gold and silver, one on the inside, and one on the outside, and covered with precious stones. We collected the gold, as well as the amulets, and the jewels that were with him, and the metal that was on his coffins. We found the queen in the same manner and collected all we could find on her. Then we set the coffins on fire. We took the furniture that we found with them, as they contained things of gold, silver, and bronze, and divided the stolen property among us . . . ."

In the following centuries the Egyptian kingdom deteriorated and foreign nations controlled the land of the Nile: Persians, Libyans, Assyrians, and Ethiopians. In 332 BC, Alexander the Great took Egypt from the Egyptians. After his death the Ptolemies inherited the land and in 30 BC it became Roman.

Egyptian culture ceased to be known until Napoleon awakened interest in it again and established the first Institute for Egyptian Research. He was a good observer and during his Egyptian campaign of 1799, he noticed many of the problems of the land:

In no land has the administration such an influence on the well being of the people. If the administration is good, channels are carefully cleaned and maintained in good condition, rules of irrigation are well executed, and the flood reaches extensive areas. When administration is poor, corrupt, or weak, canals are obstructed with mud, dams are poorly maintained, irrigation rules are not adhered to, and the bases of the irrigation system are damaged in many areas by the anti-administration position and the private interests of some people. A government has no influence on rain and snowfall in the Beause or in Brie. In Egypt, however, the government of the land has a definite influence on the extension of the watering which takes place. This makes the difference between the Egypt ruled by the Ptolemies and the present Egypt that began falling apart with the Romans and was destroyed by the Turks.

What happened to the people who again worshiped the daily returning sun as the deity Re? Their descendants still live on the shores of the Nile: they are the Copts who accepted Christianity, as taught by the apostle Mark. The Copts are the founders of one of the oldest Christian sects and their churches are still found today in all cities. However, ninety percent of the Egyptian population have their roots in the Islamic faith, resulting from the invasion of Arabic people in the seventh century AD and who conquered the entire Mideast. In AD 968 the Fatimides arrived in Egypt (they founded the University el-Azhar), and in AD 1169, the Sultan Saladin conquered the kingdom, the Mamelukes, and finally the Ottomans.

Prologue

How the Hieroglyphs
Were Rediscovered

September 27, 1822 is a significant date for egyptology and for medicine. On this date in Paris appeared a very much gaped-at Signore Belzoni, whose occupation was muscle-man and traveling entertainer. He had a wagon and load, which he decorated to a swanky display on the "Boulevard of Italy." In imitation of the tomb of the Pharaoh Sethos I (an Italian artist worked on this for twenty-seven months), there stood a sarcophagus, a number of mummies, and various imitations of Egyptian grave rubbish. The sight was pleasantly grotesque for the fine ladies. But this was not the reason for the significance of the date.

On this same sunny, autumn day, an unassuming man from the Rue Mazarine in Paris gave a certain Jean-François Champollion of the Académie of Incripitions et Belles Lettres an incomparable little book: "Lettre a l'alphabet des hiéroglyphes phonetiques." (This was supposedly followed by the subtitle "Précis du système hiéroglyphique" one year later.) All of Paris was crazy with excitement and at least the cultivated circles had their sensation. The discovery of Tutankhamun's tomb in Deir el Bahri approximately 100 years later did not cause nearly as great a sensation.

But what did the excitement have to do with the thirty-two-year-old Champollion? To answer this, we must briefly refer to Napoleon's Egyptian campaign of 1799. During this campaign, trenches were being dug at Fort Julien near Rosetta. An artillery captain named Bouchard, an unpopular, overbearing slave-driver, who would not even allow his men a cool drink in the brutal heat, led the work. One day while sitting in the shade, he observed one of his men stumble over a stone. Enraged, he began beating him. But Bouchard fell silent in the middle of the punishment when he saw the unusual characters on the stone. "Spoils of war," he assumed, and "valuable." Here he was correct.

The stone was taken to Alexandria to the house of General Menon. From there the British confiscated it in 1801, after their victory over the French, and shipped the basalt slab, which weighed tons, to their homeland. In the course of the year 1802, the "Rosetta stone" was exhibited in the British Museum in London, where it still lies today.

The text of the stone is etched in three languages on the badly damaged slab. It describes a decree of the Egyptian priests' synod, which met in Memphis to honor the young King Ptolemy V Epiphanes, dated 27 March 196 BC. What else was contained therein is not important. For the privileges protected by the temple and the Egyptian people, a series of honors were decided upon, which were also renewed later in the first Philae decree for the king and his wife Cleopatra I. Despite the fact that a copy of this stone was to be erected in every temple, another stone has not yet been found.

The text of the Rosetta stone is preserved in Greek (the last twenty-seven lines are missing), demotic characters (the first fourteen lines are missing), and in hieroglyphics. It was clear to the ambitious bookkeeper's son, Champollion, that it would be possible to key the hieroglyphics with the Greek and demotic characters.

Hieroglyphics had already been known for centuries, but since the time of the ancient Greeks, no one had been capable of deciphering them. It was therefore believed that hieroglyphics had to do with secret religious symbols and were not a true script. Scholarly individuals conducted imaginative discussions and interpretations, such as those of the German Jesuit Athanasius Kirchner (AD 1601–1680), who interpreted the simple inscription "Osiris says" in this way: "The life of things, after Typhon's conquer, the dampness of nature, through the alertness of Anubis."

Facts known to be true replaced all speculations twenty-three years after the discovery of the stone. And after that memorable day in September 1822, modern egyptology began. Grave inscriptions and chiseled temple walls were finally open books; the many papyri no longer concealed the exciting history of ancient Egypt. Researchers were no longer dependent on the posthumous works of Greek historians but could instead dive into the wondrous world of the pharaohs themselves. And such direct methods of research led to truly breathtaking insights into the great quality of ancient Egyptian medicine.

Upon the instructions of the Prussian King Frederick William IV, Fredrick Lepsius undertook the first large expedition to Egypt. Many significant scientists henceforth snatched away the secrets of the Nile in the desert; probably the most significant among the scientists was the Frenchman Auguste Mariette, who founded the Egyptian Museum in Cairo, the largest and richest museum of Egyptian culture in the world.

Sensational things have been found during the last century, which seem insignificant compared to the millennium that have passed since the days of the Egyptian advanced civilization. But many riddles about the "loved country of the gods" remain unsolved.

The Secrets
of the Papyri

*It is the power of truth
that endures!*
(Teaching of Ptahhotep, 2400 BC)

One may well ask: how do papyri—even those about medicine—which are carefully guarded and kept behind lock and key, actually look? They are not books, even though they may discuss the "Book of Eye Diseases" or "Book of Wounds." They are rolls of papyrus, which are produced today as they were 4,000 years ago. Every tourist in Egypt can see in the small factories, to which one is guided in every organized pyramid tour, how the water plants are cut into strips, laid over each other, and pressed. After approximately one week, a tight page, upon which it is possible to write and draw, is created.

The papyri of ancient times were pages approximately forty centimeters long and roughly thirty-two centimeters wide, which in mass production was sold in pieces that were eight meters long. The language in the documents that have been handed down to us is a middle Egyptian language with ancient and new Egyptian words. As in Arabic writing today, one reads the inscriptions from right to left, in columns of various widths (ranging from fifteen to twenty-seven centimeters), and to this, in horizontal lines underneath each other (eighteen to twenty-six per page). The texts of the papyri were not written in hieroglyphics but rather in what is known in Greek as "hieratic." The difference is rather like that between print and cursive scripts. It was simply faster for the writer to write "in hieratic." The titles, details about quality, and instructions for drug intake were written in red ink, the rest was in black. The papyri were inscribed on both sides.

Under the forty-two "Hermetic books" of the Egyptians, which were named by Clemens Alexandrinus in 200 BC, there were also six medical books: "About the Anatomy of the Body," "About Disease," "About the Instruments" (of the physician), "About Cures," "About Eye Diseases," and "About the Conditions of Women."

The books have been lost, hence all their contents is uncertain. Clemens did not remark about this. But what he did make note of in a few lines must have been accurate, because we also find from the historian Diodor in 50 BC a report about a holy book that was compulsory reading for Egyptian doctors. The physicians were required to have received the book from a book dealer "as they were written by numerous famous doctors of ancient times."

As one always judges these and similar reports, one can be comforted that comprehensive medical records were summarized in a systematically ordered way and codified. Probably, the greatest part of this was discovered in the meantime. The collection of texts that were found are all but systematic. They are difficult to understand. For the most part, the papyri consist of loose single texts, all-in-all, approximately 1,200.

A large part of the prescription texts are confusing to us because we cannot produce the ancient medications, due to our ignorance of many drugs. Many are naturally guessed at. For example, "When a man with *whj*-visions in his excrement chews upon from its fruit, then it reacts in an elimination of the disease in the stomach of the man." The oil contained the *dgm*-plant is meant; we assume that it is the *Recinus communis*. And it is named this way in another prescription (Papyrus Ebers no. 25), "For the emptying of the stomach, (for) the healing of a disease in the stomach of a man; fruit of the *dgm*-plant is chewed and washed down with beer, until everything that is in the stomach comes out."

The author of the medical records is unknown. In any case, the statements are correct but certainly were not recorded by a doctor as they are copies of older drafts which are up to 1,000 years old. There is no substantial evidence of a personal dictation from the doctor to the scribe, especially because the same prescriptions appear in the different papyri. That must have been a rare "quack" who did not realize that he constantly repeated himself. Presumably, amateur scribes worked for clients. And it is also probable that the scribes wanted to perfect their art with medical texts. They could have elected themes that were more full of relish: about the beauties on the Nile, for example, or the magnificence of the gold palaces. Their medical ignorance is also apparent in that a good scribe simply did not know to which body part the referred treatment belonged to. In Papyrus Ebers no. 102 and no. 296, the same treatment is given for completely different ailments.

It seems certain that the prescriptions and treatments of many unnamed physicians were written on notes, and then these single pieces of paper were later summarized in the large collected works.

Many diagnoses presumably stem back to the Old Kingdom. Despite this, it is probable that physicians also cheated a little. For example, a prescription fell directly from heaven into the courtyard of the temple of Chemmis and was "brought as a wonder to King Khufu." A pale moon, the scribe added, accompanied the scene. Other dispensings came personally from the gods. Therefore, according to the motto: for Isis from Re, highly personal.

There is a linguistic reason to support the conjecture that many medical texts are very old. The Papyrus Smith, for example, contains a complete flourish of idioms and expressions that were completely unusable at the end of the Middle and New Kingdoms. Most of the Egyptians no longer understood them. Therefore, such expressions must have been "copied" by the scribe from much earlier texts, unless the scribe still knew the original meaning of the word and commented so in the margins. For instance, in the Papyrus Smith it is written that the patient is to "stay close to his landing post." In other words, proper bedrest is recommended? Not by a longshot! Our scribe, certainly a crafty old boy, commented in this way, "The patient should be put on his regular diet and should receive no medicine."

The Egyptians' earliest medical literature consisted of monographs, which were later combined into compendiums. The contents of one of these is assumed here, because other documents about the theme were missing. It has to do with the "Veterinarian Papyrus of Kahun," a fragment that proves to us the existence of veterinary medicine. As in many other cultures, veterinary medicine developed parallel to human medicine and had great meaning, especially for farmers. The loss of an ox may have been worse to some than the death of a child, because the child was "replaceable" without cost, whereas the ox was not. We do not know anything about Egyptian veterinarians except that perhaps they were self-educated shepherds or were physicians who also cared about animals. The papyrus fragment from Kahun is mainly dedicated to dogs and bulls:

When I see a bull with gas, then his eyes water, his forehead is wrinkled, the roots of his teeth are red, his neck is swollen. Repeat the conjuration for him. Let him lie on his side and sprinkle him with cold water, let his eyes, his hoofs, and his entire body be rubbed with pumpkin and melons, let him be smoked with pumpkins...wait shepherds...soaked...so that it draws when it soaks through...until it dissolves in water. Let him be rubbed with pumpkin or cucumber....

Occasional notes about the usefulness of the prescriptions that were written in the margins of the papyri show that the great "books" of medical knowledge also had users and did not just "waste away" in the libraries. Other notes indicated such comments as "he is a senior physician, who reads the book daily" or "to him one brings a case of writings." One doctor kept himself knowledgeable with regular lectures, and his colleague took medical literature to his patients. This latter instance may have been out of carefulness because Diodor, the Hellenic historian, noted, "whenever the physician is not successful in saving the patient but exactly complies with the rules of the holy book, he is safe from any accusations. If he acted against the instructions, then the death penalty can be imposed, whereby the lawmaker begins by saying that only seldom would it occur that a few have more insight than the instructed treatments, which have been founded after many years of observation and have been compiled by the most brilliant masters." It is unknown whether any physicians would have wanted, in those days long ago, to prove an error in

medical practice; there is no evidence of any execution for this reason.

Three centuries after the deciphering of the hieroglyphs by Champollion, the scientific processing of the medical papyri began in 1853 with Heinrich Brugsch—a respectable researcher—with his essay, "The Medical Knowledge of the Ancient Egyptians and About an Ancient Egyptian Medical Manuscript in the Royal Museum in Berlin." It deals with a papyrus he found, named "Berlin 3038." But before embarking on a discussion of the papyri themselves, it might be helpful to explain that the papyri are named for the places where they are kept or for the first owner or the editor of the first publication. The medical papyri all have in common the attribute of sober observation, and the practical rules and details of treatment mentioned are completely scientific. This is also true for descriptions of "hopeless" cases, which could only have been included out of theoretical interest. The Papyrus Ebers even contains two treatments that provide evidence of the systematic scientific interest of the ancient Egyptian physicians, they are titled "The Secret of the Physicians" and "The Knowledge of the Movement of the Heart and the Knowledge of Heart." According to the latter, the human body contains forty-six "vessels," which contain mucus, blood, semen, urine, the breath of life, and the breath of death. In the "Secret of the Physicians," twenty-two vessels of the human body are mentioned, which have a connection with the limbs. They are divided into eleven pairs and were of interest to the physicians for that reason; certain illnesses were supposed to have had their origin there. The meaning of the heart and its relationship to pulse (for the Egyptians, "The heart speaks in all limbs") is mentioned correctly. They also correctly identified the function of the heart as a "pumping station" with availability of "canals to all body parts." On this theory of the heart, they based their education of the living function of the human. "They were not far from the discovery of circulation," the egyptologist J. H. Breasted wrote.

and give a prognosis of birth. The pain befalls in specific sequences: eye ailments; inability to see; neck pain; the patient smells like roasted meat; pain of the anus, intestines, base of the leg; pain in the neck and in the ears; hearing problems; pain in the genitalia and all limbs; urinary problems; insomnia; pain in the thigh; the same, but only on one side; thirst; pain in the perineum. The last section—"...you should have an affect on them..."—describes the fumigation of the genitalia, enemas, and medications to take or to massage into the legs.

The history of the papyri

The oldest papyrus

The oldest papyrus is the Papyrus Kahun. Its age can be documented because a small statement from the time of King Amenemhet III, who lived from 1840 to 1792 BC, is written on the back side. The first publication was in 1898 by F. Griffith, London, "Hieratic Papyri from Kahun and Gurob."

The Papyrus Kahun includes seventeen diagnoses about female diseases of the genitalia and seventeen single texts that mention agents that are to enable conception

Papyrus Edwin Smith

The Papyrus Smith is the "brother" to the Papyrus Ebers, as both appeared in an antique store in Thebes. Both papyri were offered as rolls, to Edwin Smith as well as to George Ebers, and this resulted in curious exchanges. Smith, who actually worked as a farmer in Upper Egypt, was extremely interested in the excavations of ancient Thebes and bought the papyrus rolls in 1862. He was an American who had studied in London, Paris, and Cairo (also Egyptian writing) but did not, however, become interested in a translation of his roll. In 1906, his daughter gave the papyrus to the New York Historical Society. Only in 1930 did the American egyptologist J. H. Breasted successfully translate the papyrus, after ten years of painstaking work. The text originated between about 3000 and 2600 BC, and a commentary with sixty-nine comments is dated back to the year 25 BC. The Papyrus Smith itself appeared about the year 1550 BC (in other sources the year of 1700 BC is given), is fifteen centimeters wide, and almost five meters long. The high quality of the medical description in Papyrus Smith is due to the lively interest of the researchers and scientists of the other papyri, who, at the turn of the century (and similar to Egyptian medicine) were treated as trivial.

The first edition of the translated papyrus was completed by James H. Breasted in 1930 in Chicago and was called "The Edwin Smith Surgical Papyrus, Published in Facsimile and Transliteration with Translation and Commentary in Two Volumes." In 1931 in volume 231 of the *German Journal of Surgery*, pages 645 to 690, Max Meyerhof reported "about the Papyrus Edwin Smith, the oldest book of surgery in the world."

On the front side of the Papyrus Smith there are seventeen columns and on the other side, five. The front side contains, with forty-eight case reports, the "Book of Wounds"; the reverse side has prescriptions.

The "Book of Wounds" is a modern choice of name. How it was titled originally, perhaps "Collections of Accidents" or something similar, is unknown, because the first column was severely damaged. The case re-

ports of wounds are given in the order of body parts, beginning with the head, neck, shoulders, arms, upper body, etc. Nevertheless, it is obvious that only a part of the original text is preserved. The Papyrus Smith stops in the middle of a sentence describing a treatment for the lower spinal cord. There is every reason to believe that the complete text also included injuries of the stomach, the pelvis, the legs, and the foot.

Max Meyerhofer wrote in 1931:

The author of the book of surgery wrote his work in a tremendously methodical manner, in that he consistently advances from the head downwards to the organs lying below. And with every body part, he proceeds from the lighter wounds of the soft body parts to the more complicated and serious fractures. At the same time, he designed his books into an educational and a correctly scholastic form. His book, in its form, is arranged for cramming and memorizing. I find similar books again in the Arabic medical literature of the middle ages, whereby the Greek translators very often wrote and methodically simplified works from Hypocrites and Galen in the form of questions and answers, in order to make the learning process for physicians as simple as possible.

Following is example case 41 of the wound book titled, "For a Malignant Wound in his Breast":

When you examine a man with a malignant wound in his breast, and this wound is infected and heat streams out of the opening of this wound against your hand, and the borders of this wound become colored, and that man has a fever....Then you should say to that one who has a malignant wound in his breast, that is infected. He has a fever. An ill-one, whom I want to treat....Then you should make him a cool medium to draw out the heat and open the wound.... Then you should make him a medium to dry the wound...make it smaller, and bind it with this. If the same happens on some other body part, then you should treat him with these instructions accordingly.

It remains to be seen which agents were used for treatment.

In twenty-two of the forty-eight cases, the patient should (only on the first day) be bound with fresh meat, in order to stop the bleeding as soon as possible. In the next days, as it was instructed in a few of the more serious cases, only a salve of fat, honey, and a material from plants was applied. The fat was to promote dampness to provide protection from the exterior. The honey drew water and acted as an antiseptic, and the respective plant materials were to contract the wound and let it heal quicker.

In the wound book, the treatment of fractures was also described in detail:

Case 25: "When you examine a man [with] a lower jaw that is displaced, and you find his mouth open, so that you cannot close his mouth; then you should put your finger [both index fingers] on the end of both the jawbones in the inside of his mouth, and put both your thumbs under his chin; then you must let them [the displaced joint bone, that is] fall together in their places... .

Bandage them with *imr·w* and honey every day, until he is better."

Case 35: "When you examine a man with a fractured clavicle, where one is shortened...then you must lay him down, stretched out, so that something domed is in between his shoulder blades; then you should make a spread on his shoulders, until his clavicles stretch out, until the fracture falls into place. Then you must make him two linen bandages; then you must put one on the inside of his arm, the other lay underneath his arm. Then you should bandage him: treat him with honey every day...."

On the other side of the Papyrus Smith there are a number of treatments for fetor, a diagnosis of a woman's disease and two beauty treatments

The plague (we assume that this is meant by *i3d·t*) must have come every year and brought disease and death: "Saying for protection against the breath of the plague of the year." (Papyrus Smith 18.1–11): "It is to be recited over an amulet."

Such sayings or magical formulas are evident in almost all of the papyri. Professor Dr Hermann Ranke gave his opinion, which is also valid today, about this in 1948 in a program aired on radio Stuttgart (part of the "University of Heidelberg Hour"):

In several cases in which human help failed, a final attempt was undertaken, from an unnatural source. In other cases, the medication was administered with magical spells or a number of prescriptions without magical spells—again, according to the discrepancy of the doctor, in case his patient expressly wanted a magical spell. If, finally, the text of Papyrus Ebers is introduced through three magical spells that were to be recited whenever one took a medication, drank a concoction, or took off a bandage, then this can be interpreted in no other way than that of an expression in the belief of the help of the gods. We cannot forget that even during the enlightened time of the Greeks in the writings of Hippocrates (upon which we swore as our patron), Apollo was called upon. And even today, good health is prayed for.

Papyrus Ebers—
the comprehensive medical
papyrus

Papyrus Ebers is used as our founding book for the knowledge of ancient Egyptian medicine. On its reverse side there is a little calendar with the dates of Sothis (Sothis = Sirius with its heliacal rising, about at the beginning of the cresting of the Nile, when the Egyptian year began) from the ninth year of King Amenophis I (1536 BC).

The egyptologist George Ebers (1837–1898) was a university professor in Leipzig. In 1873, an Arab in Luxor offered to sell him the papyrus. The seller claimed to have found it eleven years previously between the legs of a mummy. It was first published in 1875 in Leipzig in a paper titled "Papyrus Ebers. The Hermetic Book about the Medications of the Ancient Egyptians in Hieratic Writing. Published, with Summary and Introduction Included, from George Ebers.

With Hieroglyphic-Latin Glossary from L. Stern." The first really dependable translation, however, did not appear until 1937 by the Norwegian medical historian B. Ebball.

Aside from its medical diversity, the Papyrus Ebers is exceptional in its poetic language. There is, for example, a comparison made between a "wrinkled fruit" and a boil and between "fleeting breath" and unconsciousness.

The papyrus comprises 108 columns (100 on the front side), which are divided into forty-five groups. The second group, for example, describes a comprehensive collection of prescriptions, with instructions for laxatives, the regulation of defecation and urinary elimination for intestinal worms, and so forth. The majority of medications should be drunk or chewed; others are used as suppositories or enemas. In the fourth group, stomach ailments are discussed (and in a tremendously lively way). It is so vivid that one has the impression of sitting in front of an internist who is trying to find the cause of the illness and alleviate the pain. However, the texts are difficult to understand and are full of unknown expressions. The "Collected Book of the Eyes" is in the sixteenth group, where ninety-five prescriptions are summarized, and the forty-third section describes the first of the two books contained in the Papyrus Ebers about the heart and the circulatory system: "The Secret of the Heart."

Such minor ailments as, for example, a cough are only mentioned briefly in the Papyrus Ebers. There is a short prescription in the Papyrus Ebers that is also in the Papyrus Berlin in a longer version. It is explained similar to the following but in more detail: pieces of plant and mineral substances should be heated on hot stones. A pot with a hole bored into it should be put on top of this and a pipe should be put into the hole. The patient must "swallow" the herbal steam seven times. And because the mouth dries out, it should be rinsed out with oil. ("Swallowing" meant inhaling. In the Egyptian Arabic manner of speech, Egyptians also "drink" their tobacco today!)

Papyrus Hearst

The Papyrus Hearst was unearthed in the Dair-al-Ballas (Upper Egypt) by an Arab. It is so named for Mrs Phoebe Hearst, who bequeathed it to the University of California. About one third of the Ebers' text is also found in the Hearst papyrus. It is seventeen centimeters high and three and a half meters long and is dated earlier than the Papyrus Ebers. Once again, it was first published in Leipzig in 1905 as "The Hearst Medical Papyrus. Hieratic Text in 17 Facsimile Plates in Collotype with Introduction and Vocabulary by George A. Reisner."

Papyrus Berlin

Heinrich Brugsch found the Papyrus Berlin several meters deep in the ground, in a vessel, while excavating in Saqqara. The papyrus is from about 1300 BC with numerous orthographic errors. It is twenty centimeters high and a little over five meters long. It awakened the interest of the public in Leipzig. In 1863 Heinrich Brugsch wrote "Recueil de monuments égyptiens," Volume II. The Papyrus Berlin is richer and more interesting than the Papyrus Hearst. The Papyrus Ebers and Papyrus Berlin have similar concluding statements in the notes of the circulatory book, "it is the vessels of the legs that begin to die off." In Papyrus Berlin, six prescriptions are added that are purportedly from a doctor named Neterhotep.

Papyrus Beatty VI

The Papyrus Beatty VI deals, first of all, with diseases of the anus. The beginning and the end of the papyrus are quite damaged. It is twenty-one centimeters wide and a little over one meter long. The first edition was published in London in 1935 by Alan H. Gardiner: "Hieratic Papyri in the British Museum. Third Series: Chester Beatty Gift."

Papyrus London

This papyrus, with its few original prescriptions and its many magical spells, borders between medicine and magic. It was recorded in 1350 BC, is seventeen centimeters wide and just over two meters long. The beginning and end of the papyrus are broken off. Its first publication was in Leipzig in 1912 by W. Wreszinski: "The London Medical Papyrus."

Papyrus Carlsberg VIII

This has been preserved only in pieces ten centimeters wide. Three columns are readable. The essays were recorded about 1200 BC. It was published in 1939 by Erik Iversen in Copenhagen: "Papyrus Carlsberg No. VIII with some Remarks on the Egyptian Origin of some Popular Birth Prognoses."

Contents of the papyri
(According to the classification of Prof Grapow)

In general. Medication for fever; prescription book for the uses of the *dgm*-plant; drugs to drink after taking any medication; "sayings" to accompany this.

Injuries and wounds. Diagnosis of the wound book; recipes for broken bones; impact wounds; burns; bites.

Growths, swelling, itching. Diagnoses and prescriptions for different types of growths; prescriptions for the treatment of swelling and itching.

Ailments of the head. General prescriptions; prescriptions for eye ailments; earaches, the nose, and the mouth (for tongue and teeth).

Ailments of the limbs. Prescriptions for ailments of the fingers and toes; prescriptions for leg pain.

Diseases of the internal organs. General prescriptions to stimulate appetite and digestion; prescriptions for different types of ailments—stomach ailments (diagnoses and prescriptions); prescriptions for ailments of the heart, lungs, and liver; ailments of the anus and bladder.

Respiratory illnesses. Prescriptions for cough; diagnoses and prescriptions for 'st·t (rheumatism?).

Women's ailments. Actual women's ailments; prescriptions for the female breast; prognoses of birth and other.

Beauty treatments. Beauty treatments; prescriptions for hair care.

Household products. Prescriptions for smoking mechanisms; prescriptions for the prevention of pests.

Drawings of doctors; surgical tools. Physician; senior physician; priest (the sachmet); magician; well-informed one—lecturing priest; subordinate of the physician—bandager; shepherd (veterinarian to cattle).

Instruments. Set of instruments (of the doctor) found in an emergency bag:

Rush (used as a knife for cutting treatments).
Fire drill (to burn growths).
Knife/chisel (to open the mouth).
Cupping glass.
Curcurbitulae.
Thorn (to burst a burn blister).
hnw: instrument to pack a growth and its contents.
hmm: instrument to burn a growth ("if using a knife, warm it in a fire, then the wound will not bleed so much" (Papyrus Ebers no. 872). "When it bleeds a lot, you should burn it with fire" (Papyrus Ebers no. 876). "But be careful of the vessels (Papyrus Ebers nos. 860 and 871).
Heated broken glass, for eye treatments.
Swabs, tampons, linen material.
Normal knives, salve spoons, mortars, etc.

One can only imagine how enemas were administered. Maybe with a horn that had an opening on the point, such as can be seen in the Louvre in Paris. The instruction "pour in with a vulture feather" probably meant to use a hollow feather quill like a pipette. We are not certain about treatments in hospitals; they could have been connected with schools. As a rule, one treated patients on the spot.

Diagnoses

The diagnoses in the papyri have no rigid scheme but are developed along the following five points:

1. For the title, they all have this in common (in contrast to the medication, where drinks, salves, or powders are written): *š's3·w*, actually meant "Instructions for Recognition and Treatment (of an illness)."

2. The formula "When you examine ..." is actually translated as "when you do without, weigh" or "when you test" (namely the growths, which are partly removable by surgery). (Papyrus Ebers no. 436: "When you examine a bite of a crocodile . . . .") The examination (inspection) was successful by questioning, probing with the hands and fingers ("palpation"), and smelling. Hearing was not used as an aid by the ancient Egyptians. Percussion (knocking in order to recognize a difference in the sound) was as unknown as auscultation (listening for unnatural sounds). In its place, one observed the stool; patients with stomach ailments would lie on their backs while they were examined by the doctor.

3. The formula "You should say . . . ." In a section of the treatment introduced as such, the doctor decides the type of illness. It is successful in the form of the sentence "this is the illness so and so." Then the degree of chance of healing follows. What occurs very seldom, mind you, is "it is a hopeless case."

4. The formula "You should

make..." the part of treatment. In-struction of a prescription or details about a bandage, etc, are described.

5. The text of the papyri employs interesting similies. For instance, it is described how a palpating finger causes an indentation on the stomach, which then evens out again; "it [the stomach] goes and comes under your fingers like oil in a hose" (Papyrus Ebers no. 199). In another case, a patient received an agent that is eliminated through the mouth or the anus inclusively; "it looks like the blood of a pig after it is heated." A growth on the head is described as "pointed and raised like a female breast." In the book of wound injuries, a head injury is compared with the fontanelle of a child (Papyrus Smith, case 8):

When you examine a man with a gaping wound on his head, that reaches the bone, the skull is splintered, the brain of his skull is broken open; then you should palpate the wound, and you find the break that is on his skull is like those wrinkles that form on poured metal; there is something inside that trembles [and] flutters under your fingers like the weak part of the top of the skull of a child that has not yet become solid. A trembling and fluttering under your fingers develops as soon as the brain of the skull is broken open. Blood comes out of the nostrils; the patient suffers from stiffness to his neck. Then you should say: this may not be treated.

There is a note written in the margin, "[This is] a large splinter that is open to the inside of his skull, [namely] the skin, that surrounds his brain; and this is how it is broken open [and] pours out of the inside of his head." The excretion that is described in the course of this extensive text could be the "liquor cerebrospinalis" (brain-spinal cord fluid). With the most varied ailments of the brain, the fluid of the spinal cord gives the most valuable diagnostic indications. It is possible that the ancient Egyptian doctors knew this.

When the prognosis is bad and the patient will barely survive, the goal of therapy is simply to wait, "you should brush the wound with fat, you should not bandage it, you should not fasten two strips onto it, until you know that he has reached a decided point...." Exact observations and descriptions provide us with numerous other cases that the ancient physicians diagnosed just as quickly as do their colleagues today, for example, risus sardonicus (a fixed smile and elevated eyebrows resulting from tetanus), aphasia (speech impediments resulting from brain injuries), or hemiplegia (a motor disability of one side of the body).

These are amazing findings from the medicine of the pharaohs, 1,000 years before Homer allowed his Iliad to be recited, "a doctor is to be regarded as higher than many others because he cuts out arrows and scatters relieving herbs."

Obviously the ancient physicians could do much more: a picture from antiquity (First and Second Dynasties) apparently shows a tracheotomy, the surgical opening of the

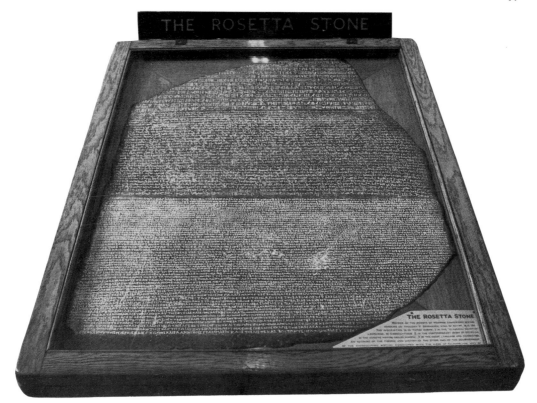

THE ROSETTA STONE

This piece of stone marked the beginning of unraveling ancient Egyptian writing. In 1799, a French captain tripped over it during bulwark work at Fort Julian at Rosetta. In 1802 the stone was sent, together with other amazing writings, as war booty to England. It is still there today, on exhibit in London. In the Rosetta stone is chiseled a decree of the Egyptian priests' synod. It was done in March 196 BC in three languages: Greek, demotic, and hieroglyphics. With the aid of the Greek text it was possible to translate the Egyptian text. Twenty-three years after the discovery of the stone, the Frenchman Jean Francois Champollion was able to solve the riddle of the hieroglyphs. Only then did modern archaeology start: tomb script and chiseled walls of temples finally became "open books," and the many papyri did not occult any further the exciting history of ancient Egypt. *British Museum, London.*

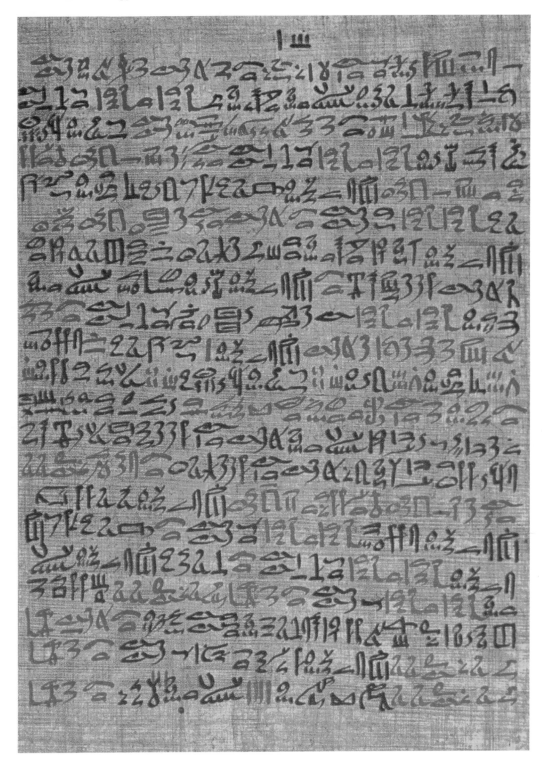

Opposite page: Part of the all-encompassing medical text of the Papyrus Ebers. The papyrus is twenty meters long, was found in 1862, and had been written in 1536 BC, in hieratic—a short form of hieroglyphics. *Facsimile; German Medicine Historical Museum, Ingolstadt.*

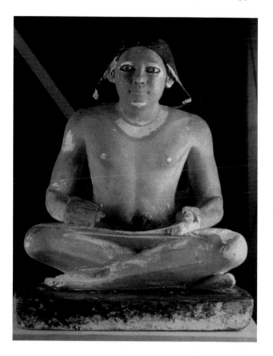

Right: This plaster statue of a scribe with papyrus roll comes from the time of the Fourth/Fifth Dynasty (Old Kingdom, 2600–2190 BC). The medical papyri, however, were put together many centuries later, enlarged, and copied. In part they appeared in "note collections" with recipes, drug information, and treatment modalities that were already 1,000 years old. *Egyptian Museum, Cairo.*

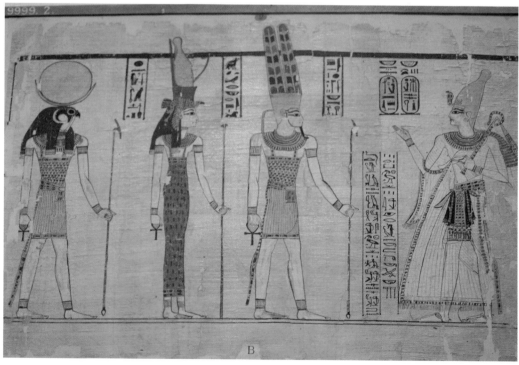

This papyrus was prepared about 400 BC and shows the "Triad of Thebes": a pharaoh asks the gods Khons, Nut, and Amun for welfare. *British Museum, London.*

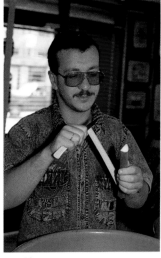
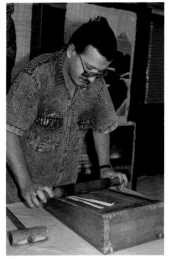
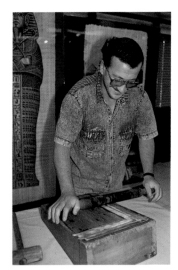
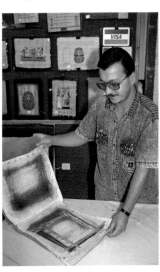
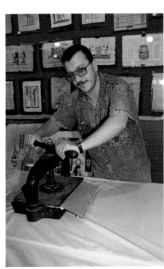
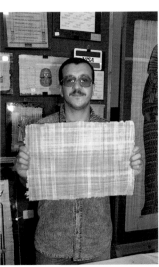

Only a few minutes from the pyramids in Giza there are several stores in which papyri are prepared, written, and painted according to old patterns. The preparation is done just as it was for centuries. The water plant is grown in ponds, its stalk is then cut in strips that are placed parallel and cross-wise over each other. After a week in a press, the strips have formed a strong "paper." The papyri of ancient times were leaves about forty centimeters long and about thirty-two centimeters wide that were fabricated and brought into commerce in pieces about eight meters long. The language that we received is from Middle Egypt, with some terms from the ancient and some new Egyptian mixed in. The writing was done—as it still is in Arabic—from right to left.

airway above and below the thyroid in cases of choking. And in the Anatomical Museum of Cairo there are three skulls with very smooth margins of circular holes, a clear indication of "trephination" (opening of the skull).

About the prescriptions

The number of prescriptions is very great: about 900 are known to us, but these are by far not all that there were. If we limit ourselves to the most important, the prescriptions of Papyrus Ebers build the best foundations.

Special Instructions

phr·t = medication (ie, bandage, drink, or salve).

hr- = liquid medication (sweet fruit juice with water).

swrj·t = drink (only for stomach ailments).

mrh = oil drink.

gś·w = salve.

'sdm = makeup (this is found infrequently, under the prescriptions for eye ailments. Only a single prescription gives improved sight as a reason for the makeup.) Egyptian doctors assigned cosmetics to the medical field. The Papyrus Ebers, for example, contains the following recipe for wrinkles: one grinds a portion of pistachio tree, wax, fresh Behen-oil (from the Moringe, a plant similar to the poppy), and Cyprus grass, mixes it in plant juice and rubs it onto one's face daily. For dry skin, the following is recommended: mix gall bladder of the cow, oil, rubber, and flour of the ostrich plume. This should be thinned with plant oil and the face should be washed with this daily.

tmtw = "scattering elements" (powder). There are three types of these prescribed medications. They are effective for drying wounds or drying a "running" ear.

mt = suppositories. There are several prescriptions whose medications are to be administered in the form of a suppository.

kȝp·t = agents against smoke. There are two types of agents in Papyrus Ebers. One is to improve odor in the house or in clothes (ie, is not medical), the other is for pest prevention.

The prescriptions are described quite differently: some are short, some are long. Many instructions of preparation and use are abbreviated because they were probably self-explanatory for the ancient Egyptians, but this lack of detailed explanation provides difficulties for us. Examples of the shortened form: "Snake fat; used as a salve." For burn blisters on the first day, "honey is to be used in the bandage." To prevent infection, "a frog is cooked in fat; used as a salve." For the vessels, "milk of a woman that gave birth to a son; leave overnight in a new pot" ("new" probably meant clean) "until the respective cream builds; all painful

41

areas are rubbed with this." This prescription is found in other places with the additional ingredients of rubber and ram's hair. For the injured eye, "gall bladder of a pig, divided in two is to be used as makeup at night; and then half is dried and rubbed finely, and the eye is to be made up in the morning." (Papyrus Ebers no. 392–61).

Preparation of agents was usually easy. However, about forty recipes that are written in more detail point to the fact that more complicated instructions were hidden behind the simple directives "make as mass of" or "cook." Recipe number twenty-one in the Papyrus Smith consists of only one drug, a fruit that is unknown to us. It describes an agent that removes age marks on the head, hands, and the body: one takes in addition to this a large mass of the fruit, crushes it, and sets it out in the sun. After it has dried, it is shelled and cut into cubes. The fruit and the chaff are separated and mixed with water to make a soft mass that is cooked thoroughly, until it is almost solid. The cooled mass is washed in running water until the water tastes neither salty nor bitter. Again it is set out into the sun, ground up, newly mixed with water, and stirred into a paste and cooked. Oil builds on the surface, which is scooped off and may be collected in a pot, which has been rubbed with a fine clay. Only later would it be poured into a salve container. This is quite a lengthy process for a medication that only has one ingredient. We can only imagine how complicated the prescription in Papyrus Ebers no. 663 must have been; it had thirty-seven different drugs crushed together, yet the instructions are simply, "this is to be made into a mass that is to be used in a bandage."

Some medications were to be taken in "finger warmth," ie, as warm as a finger can tolerate (Papyrus Ebers no. 23) or in "pleasant warmth" (Papyrus Ebers no. 91) or "between both warmths," which probably meant lukewarm. Papyrus Hearst no. 45 has the following prescription: it consists of four drugs, one of which is honey. It does not say how it is prepared, but in the end of the direction it says it is taken for four days and "you should drop in the honey before you take it away." It does not take a Sherlock Holmes to realize that taking the pot away from the fire is the only thing that can be meant; therefore, the medicine is cooked. Beyond that, the sweetener must be added shortly before ingestion, ie, not cooked with the mixture.

Instructions for drugs

The realm of materials that are categorized as "drugs" is unlimited and includes animals, plants, minerals, food, drinks, and different parts of the human body. Approximately seventy animals are mentioned: about twenty mammals, twenty birds, ten fish, ten reptiles, insects (even unidentified ones), twenty-five plants, and twenty minerals. Of animals and plants, the following are used: meat, fat, blood, excrement, leaves, fruit, and even sawdust.

There are numerous treatments in the papyri which cannot be used medically. A salad with a dandelion leaf surely does not have the real dandelion. In ancient Egypt, the use of a "snake cabbage" plant was common, described as "growing on the stomach with white leaves" and "blossoms like lotus." However, we do not currently know of such a plant, nor do we know of a "mouse tail," "donkey head," or "feather of the Thoth" (a god). What is most interesting is the "tooth of the pond." The Coptic apothecary knows of a medicine called "tongue of the sea" (lăs-ĕn-jŏm). For The Egyptians this expression does not mean the sea or ocean, but rather the "artificial sea," the pond. In Arabic, which has taken over the Coptic expression, this means the back part of the octopus, which is used for eye ailments. The Egyptian "tongue of the pond" is, however, not found in any prescription for the eyes. Other undecipherable terms are the "coal of the wall" (maybe wood coals?), the "calcium of the oven," and the "tadpole of the canal."

Numerous Greek, Roman, and ancient German texts read like translations of Egyptian. For instance there was a saying: urine of a pregnant one is poured over wheat and barley. If the barley shoots first, then a boy will be born; if the wheat shoots first, it will be a girl. There is also a German saying (in Paullini J. *Neuvermehrte heilsame Dreckapotheke.* 4th ed. Frankfurt/M, 1713.): "make two holes in the earth, throw the barley and the other grain in, pour the pregnant one's urine in both. If the wheat shoots before the barley, then you will have a son; if, however, the barley shoots first, then you can expect a daughter." In Egyptian, the word barley is of masculine gender and wheat feminine; in German it is the opposite. The results of these urinous decisions of sex has nothing to do with magic, rather—unfortunately—only with grammar.

How an Illness Develops

My heart became weak,
my spirit was not happy
in my love.
(Sinuhe, 1970 BC)

In ancient Egypt, it was thought that illnesses were influenced by gods, especially the messengers of Sachmet, demons, or the spooking dead. They could also be conjured up by magic and could be forced into a person through the breath of a god, demon, or magician. The openings in the left side of the body were said to be most susceptible because this was the "deadly" side. Several diseases (ailments of the heart and stomach) were explained by "poison-seeds" that had been implanted into victims at night. This was deemed a sin against the laws of a god and was promptly punishable.

According to the accounts of Herodotus, physicians thought there were nutritional causes for internal illnesses:

The Egyptians use laxatives three days in a row every month and care for their health through vomit inducers and enemas, because they are of the opinion that all human illnesses originate from enjoyed meals. Therefore, it is harmful to eat the fruit of the sycamore tree. A stomach ailment can be attributed to the consumption of sharply fried or possibly spoiled meat. The victim should begin eating again when he has an appetite, and the woman should remain hungry with "particular" illnesses. If one dreams of warm beer, it is a bad dream because warm beer causes ailments, and whoever drinks water while eating a certain type of fish will get a fever.

Also according to the views of the ancient Egyptians, improperly digested food and food that was left in the body changed into harmful materials, the "pain and slime materials" that spread over the entire body and its vessels caused local ailments. Therefore, poor nutrition was the reason for infections, swelling, constipation, or stiffening. It did not matter if the food was incorrectly prepared or incorrectly combined with other foods. But, because of this, regulated defecation stood as a part of the "eternal spirituality," and the "proctologist," who had the title of "Shepherd of the Anus," belonged to the most socially acceptable specialists. The historian Diodorus wrote, "They say that there is something about the digestion of every enjoyed meal, that is excessive, and this is how diseases originate."

A Russian saying goes, "Eat until you're half-satiated, drink until you're half-drunk, then you will live completely." In the Orient, it is said, "Drink a third, eat a third, leave a third empty." And in Egypt, "We live from a quarter of what we eat, and the doctors live from the rest."

The symptoms that occurred in the duration of a disease were explained naturally: body and soul brought about disturbances reciprocally. For instance, aggravation and rage led to heart conditions; the other extreme, constipation, led to frightful visions. The Greek teaching of excretions, "Perittoma," can be traced back in the school of Knidos to the Egyptian idea of "wechedu," the disease-inducing substances that originate in the feces and reach the blood vessels. The question is whether the development of a metastasized sepsis ("pyemia") could be denoted here. Borderline cases are diseases that establish themselves due to natural and supernatural causes, such as the annual epidemic that occurs during flooding of the Nile, and which are even blamed on demons.

How a sick person feels has great (even dramaturgical) meaning in all ancient Egyptian fairy tales and legends. Sinuhe, the Egyptian who is famous worldwide because of the Hollywood film "Sinuhe, the Egyptian," tells in his memoirs about an experience that he had as he was being received by the king, "I was stretched out on my stomach, I didn't know that I lay before him, as the king greeted me in a friendly manner. I was like a man possessed by the dusk. My soul had gone. My body had become weak. My heart was in my stomach. I had, however, more awareness of life than of death; because then I heard the king's voice."

The physician, Sinuhe, participated in a campaign of the Middle Kingdom, during the last reigning year of King Amenemhet I (Twelfth Dynasty, 1991–1971 BC). When he discovered the murder of the king, he believed himself to be an accessory and fled to Syria. There Sinuhe was advanced to a tribal prince; but the closer he came to the end of his life, the more he wanted to return to his homeland. Senwosret I (1971–1929 BC), the son of Amenemhet I, discovered Sinuhe's place of residence and asked him to return to the king's court. The former internal physician of the palace returned home, was given a house with servants, and a magnificent grave. Whether or not this actually did happen is controversial. It is certain, however, that the oldest accounts of the Sinuhe story date back to the end of the Middle Kingdom. The most important papyri of this time are presently preserved in Berlin. We also know of Sinuhe texts from clay remains (also known as ostraca) and from inscriptions dating to the New Kingdom.

There is a vivid description of the poisoning of Isis, the sun god, who let himself be stung by a scorpion. After he was stung, he screamed and could not even answer Isis ("...he couldn't find his mouth to answer, as his lips quivered and all his limbs were crushed..."). When he forced himself to speak, he said, "I never had anything so painful as this, there is nothing as dangerous as this. It is not fire, it is also not water. My heart has heat. My body trembles. All my limbs have frostbite. I am colder than water, I am hotter than fire. My entire body is covered with my sweat. My eyes quiver without standing still.

I can't see clearly. The sky rains on my face" [ie, he sweats] "in the middle of the dry season...." The story ends with his salvation, "I burned the poison with heating and was stronger than flame and fire, until Isis entranced it...."

A letter describing the illness of the painter Pai reads thusly: "The painter Pai says to his son, the painter Prahotep: don't desert me, I am not well. Don't stop crying for me, because I am in the dark. My master Amun has turned away from me. Bring me some honey for my eyes and also ... real *stibium*. Do it, do it! Am I not your father? If I look for my eyes, then they are not here...."

Ancient Egyptian physicians' knowledge of anatomy

Although ancient Egyptian doctors had the opportunity to study the human body closely prior to mummification and its preparation, they did not do so, probably because of religious modesty. They therefore performed the embalming rites in moderation in order to prevent endangering the continued life of the deceased into the next kingdom. This is why exact accounts are, every now and then, integrated with fantastic ones, and why some well-founded empirical evidence is sometimes also based on religious theories. We have already seen an attempt to arrange body parts into a distinct order in the listings of the Papyrus Smith. This traditional order is presumably derived from the old death cult in which the ritual assembling of the corpse and the idolization of single body parts were a predecessor to the correctly functional preservation of the body in the hereafter. This dates back to the legend of Osiris.

Several versions of this story exist. The most-circulated one is that of the philospher and historian Plutarch (46-120 BC). For him, Osiris was the son of Geb, the earth father, and of Nut, the one who created the heavenly sky; he was the brother of Isis, Nephthys, and Seth. Peace and good fortune reigned in Egypt during the time that he—with his sister Isis as his wife—reigned over the country. But Seth was plagued with jealousy. He invited his brother to a banquet in which seventy-two conspirators participated. During the meal, Seth presented a richly jeweled trunk that he had secretly made according to Osiris' measurements. The person who could fit into the trunk was to keep it as a gift. No one accepted this offer except Osiris. As he lay in the trunk, the conspirators threw the lid on the trunk, nailed it shut, and sank it in the Nile. Confused, Isis searched for her husband until she finally found him on the bank of the river Byblos. She brought Osiris' body back to the Nile delta, but, even there, Seth discovered him again, dismembered him, and scattered the limbs of his brother throughout all of Egypt.

Once again, Isis prepared to "reassemble" her loved one. She found all the parts, except a limb of Osiris' that had been devoured by a fish. Plutarch's story ends suddenly. However, in the ancient Egyptian writings we read how it continued. The sun god, Re, personally sent Anubis (later to be named guard of embalming; during the ceremony, priests wore the jackal head of the god) from heaven. Anubis was able to completely reassemble the body and wrapped it in his skin. This is the image of Osiris that we have according to the ancient accounts: with crossed arms, wrapped in a shroud, born the second time, certainly not ruler of the earth any more, but ruler in the hereafter. In other words, the very first mummy!

According to Hermann Grapow, the anatomical knowledge of the ancient Egyptian doctors is roughly outlined with the following characteristics. Head with face and scalp. On the scalp, vertex and back of the head, covered with skin of the head and hair. In the skull, under the two parietal bones lies a brain, which is covered by the meninges. The skull bones are connected by sutures. In the head, there are seven holes for eyes, ears, nasal passages, and mouth. The face with forehead and temple, cheeks and chin; the ear with inner ear and ear lobes; the eye, that has grown to its roots, shows the black and white as well as the pupils and is equipped with brows and eyelashes; the nose, which is lifted out of the indentation of the face, stands out due to the nasal septum, which separates the nasal cavity with the two turbinate bodies from the nostrils. Under the eye, behind the ear, lies the cheekbone, in which the lower jaw is hooked, which, together with the upper jaw forms the mouth, on which the upper and lower lip, which are differentiated by teeth, which sit on roots, and the tongue. The neck contains the throat in the front, with the trachea and esophagus in the back. The nape, with seven cervical vertebrae, sits on the spine, which is composed of the vertebrae.

The arm with upper arm and under arm, hand with the back of the hand and with thumb and fingers is attached to the shoulders, which is composed of the shoulder blade and the collarbone, that pushes on the sternum in the front. The ribs sit between the spine and the sternum.

The breast with the nipples and the stomach with the navel and the abdomen, together with the sides and the back, encircle the entrails: the lungs and heart, stomach and gall bladder, liver, spleen, intestines with the rectum, and the bladder. The buttocks with the anus and the genitals, the penis of the man with foreskin and testicles, the female pudenda with the labia of the vagina and the uterus.

On the leg there is differentiation between upper leg and lower leg, with shin and calf; knee with knee cap; foot with the instep and sole, including toes.

All in all, the descriptions in the original text are a little unclear, which is probably sometimes due to inadequate knowledge of the interrelation of body parts. Therefore, no differentiation is made between vein and artery or tendon and muscle. And the word *šsb* is used for the trachea as well as for the esophagus.

May the Heart be Happy
Medical Life in Egypt

*My spouse, my brother
my friend! Don't be tired of
food, drink, noise, lust.*
(Quotation from a grave in the
Valley of the Queens)

All wishes for life of the ancient Egyptians revolve around a life filled with vitality, freshness, good health, and a death just as vital. Good health means "well-being." *"snb"* wrote the knowledgeable person in letters, which meant "stay healthy" or "live well." In a fairy tale, a prince speaks with an old man whom he comes across lying down and says: "it is your state of health, like one who lives with old age before him, who sleeps until the break of day, free from sorrow, without panting cough."

ndm = pleasant—this then is how the ancient Egyptian felt. Written in the Papyrus Ebers are the words:

I need to eat with my mouth, to empty with my anus, I must be able to drink and to have sex. May the heart be happy, may the limbs be in unscathed condition, may the neck be solid under the head, the eyes see far away, the nose breathe the air freely, the ear stay open and may it hear, the mouth open and know to answer, may the arms function and may they carry out work. It is the heart that begets every recognition, and it is the tongue that repeats what is thought in the heart. May the heart and tongue have power over all my limbs.

In the 3,000 years before Mena and until the Ptolemaics, ancient Egyptian medicine reached such a high level of recognition that foreign monarchs only asked for one thing of the pharaohs during times of peace: a physician for their court. In Homer's *Odyssey* it is written that "the Egyptians leave the entire world behind them when it comes to medicine." And: "See, as healing as this was the artistically prepared desert / which Helena, once the wife of Thon, Polydamnas / Presented in Agyptos. There the fruitful earth produces / Several juices, to good or harmful mixture. / There every one is a doctor and surpasses experience / All people; because they are indeed of the gender of Päeon."

Many physicians played a significant role in the courts of the pharaohs and were looked upon favorably by their rulers, as their titles express effusively. Take, for example, the physician Penthu, who practiced at the time of Akhenaten (Eighteenth Dynasty). He was called "Priest Atons, who has entrance and exit and uninhibited access to the king." This title is noteworthy because one first had to be able to pass the palace guards without being stopped. Penthu's high rank is also recognized by his seal: his name in hieroglyphics follows a man with a flail—a symbol of power. Over another doctor there is the title: "He was head of the priests of the Sakhmet [the lion-headed powerful one who also had his messenger send the fetor], master of the magicians, head physician of the king, who reads the book daily . . . who lays his hand on the patient at the same time he comes to know him; skillful in examination . . . ."

The court physicians were magnificently buried, and statues of them were erected so that those still living were compelled to recognize them as being above average—even above the poor doctors. In 1926, the German Hermann Junker found, in Giza, an informative stele the size of a door. His discovery near an aristocrat's grave area of the pyramids (its age could be dated about 2723 to 2563 BC) is testimony to the reputation of "Irj," the first doctor in history. The grave stone indicates that the doctor was "head of all court physicians" and "eye doctor of the palace, doctor of the body, who knows the inner juices of the body, shepherd of the king's anus, that prepares the *bm*" (unknown meaning).

In those days, the king's anus required as much care as in Molière's time. The Papyrus Chester Beatty provides an ancient Egyptian handbook for the "shepherds" or "guards of the anus."

Just as there was ranking of kings, there was also ranking of doctors; in ascending order: the "average" doctor, the head of physicians, the supervisor of physicians, and the head supervisor. In the palace, the different doctors had their head doctor, and leading them all was the "highest doctor of Upper and Lower Egypt." This title was found in inscriptions until the Thirtieth Dynasty. Logically, an ambitious doctor strove to obtain a position with the pharaoh that would ensure him gold, women, slaves, roasted geese, and full jugs of wine. In addition, doctors owned their own boats, or were rowed or sailed to wherever they were needed—or for leisure.

But even noble and high-ranking persons, the aristocratic land owners and rulers of provinces, had, in addition to their serfs in the household or work place, permanent internal physicians. Physicians who did not attain this level treated the public in temples or practiced medicine according to the instruction of the pharaoh on the giant military troops. In Sinai, physicians were needed for the copper and turquoise mines or by the temple, street, and pyramid construction sites.

All people, from the belt maker to the bordello manager, called the doctor the "knower of secret art." His "books" (ie, the papyri) contained the "secret knowledge of the physicians" and were only available to professionals who knew about the "recipes for secret drugs, as only a physician makes."

The doctor on the Nile had a title of *swnw* at that time, or *wt swnw* (head physician). Because only a few patients could read, the characters for "arrow" were enclosed with the letters; some historians suggest the reason being is that the doctor punctured growths with an arrow. A more accurate explanation would be one found from the Middle Ages, called a "disease arrow" in many descriptions. For example, St Sabastian's statue was always "larded" with arrows. (Sabastian was the patron saint of epidemics like the plague.) Figuratively, one could combine: arrow = messenger of death = physician = helper in times of need.

It was a family tradition in ancient Egypt to become a doctor. It is not certain whether positions were inherited, but fathers who were doctors wanted to pass their knowledge to their sons (as an "inheritance"). This parallels Jewish doctors who took much from Egyptian medicine. Until well into the seventeeth century there were many Jewish physician dynasties. They occurred not only because of tradition, but also because boys learned from their forefathers: Jewish students were not allowed to attend institutions of higher education.

There is no clear written evidence as to how education of doctors was handed down. In a few places, (Deir el-Medina, the Ramesseum, Muttempel in Karnak, and the grave of Ptahhotep in Saqqara) "school classrooms" have been archaeologically excavated and determined. The doctor Imhotep, who was made a god, was supposed to have founded, in Memphis, a medical school that was affiliated with a gigantic library. It still existed during Roman times and through it, European medicine acquired numerous

Egyptian healing methods and prescriptions.

The "Writer of the King and Head Physician of the Master" Uzahor-resinet reports in his autobiography (H. Schäfer, "Wiedereinrichtung einer Ärzteschule in Sais." *Gardiner Journal*, 1933:24):

His majesty, King Darius, ordered me, at the time his majesty was in Elam as the great king of all lands and highest ruler of Egypt, to come to Egypt, to equip the hall of the house of life ... after it had been destroyed. The barbarians brought me from country to country and took me to Egypt, as the king had ordered it .... I did as his majesty had ordered. I filled them [both houses] with students, consisting of the sons of influential men ... sons of poor people were not among them. I equipped them with all their personnel. I put learned men under their control. I gave them every wise man to keep ... for all their work. His majesty ordered to give them all good things, so that they could do their work. I equipped them with everything that was useful to them and every need with all their instruments, so that it was like the time in theirs [the houses]. This his majesty did, because he knew the importance of their art, and, in order to save the life of every sick one and the names of all gods, to establish their temples and their income, so that their holidays can be celebrated eternally.

Although these documents stem from the sixth century BC, it is certain that medical schools existed much earlier, and also that surgery was taught, because the teachers and students received "all their instruments." The fact that these schools were usually connected to temples should not confuse or lead us to assume that medical education had limited itself to the magical-religious. Certainly magic (covered later) plays a significant role, but the temples were, above all in the New Kingdom, the center of not only theology but also science around the world. Similarly, during the Middle Ages, cathedral schools were forerunners of universities.

We can only imagine what transpired in the medical schools. One part of Papyrus Ebers indicates that "Thoth is the leader who allows the writings to be read, who made the collected medical books, who lends knowledge to the learned ones to the doctors, who are in his employ...." It is not written how the doctors are paid for their work. The Sicilian scribe Diodor reports, "During campaigns and on trips within their boundaries, all were treated without compensation. Because they [the doctors] receive a salary from the government...." But the head physicians of the pharaoh and the "directors" of the school surely must have received a salary. The Egyptologist Henry Sigerist believes there was a type of "minister of health." Logically then, such was an official with a stable salary. Also, many "factory doctors" who practiced at the construction sites of the pyramids (360,000 people had to be treated in Giza alone) were, no doubt, paid by the pharaoh.

The general doctor, who often learned surgical techniques at the front during a war, traveled across the country because the largest part of the population did not live in cities. He was probably paid with wine and dried meat, a holy statue, or a gold ring—according to the people's means.

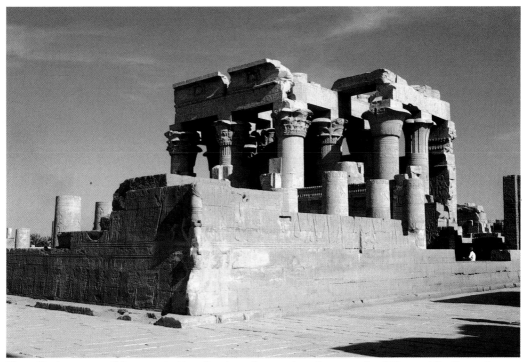

Kom Ombo—one of the most attractive temple constructions on the Nile, not far from Aswan. Tuthmosis III started the construction, the Ptolemaic Dynasty continued construction, and finally Caracalla (AD 211) finished it. The temple shows in one corridor *(below)* unique Egyptian medical representations.

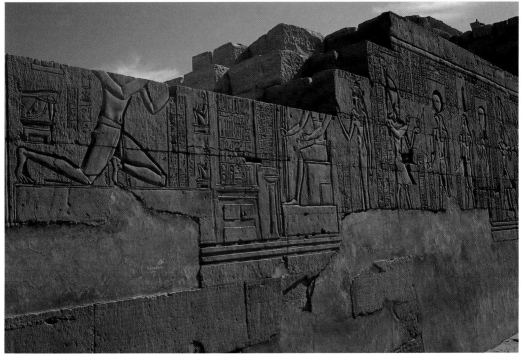

Usually not seen by tourists: a detail from the north wall of Kom Ombo. In the wall are figures of the surgical instruments commonly used.

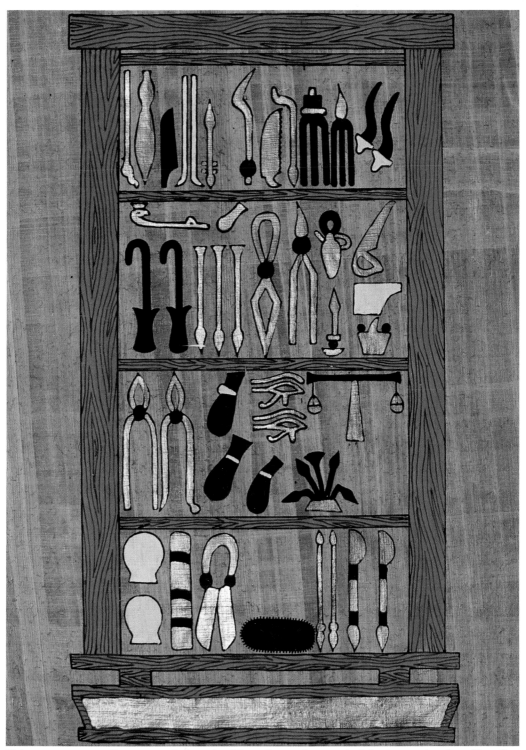

This new papyrus, from a workplace in Giza, shows the surgical instruments of an Egyptian physician according to the relief from Kom Ombo.

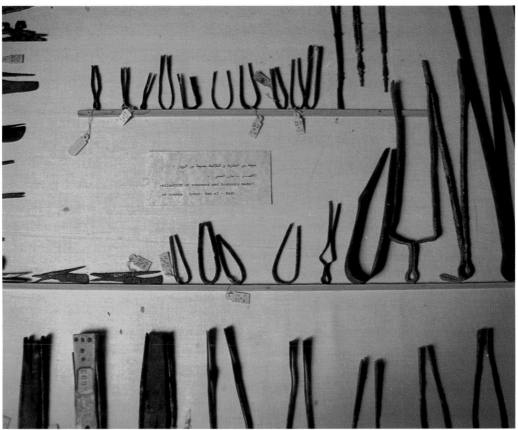

Everyone who goes up the stairs of the Egyptian Museum in Cairo to the first floor will see the room with the tomb treasures from Pharaoh Tutankhamun: the king's and the priest's coffins, household effects, utensils, chariot, and jewelry. Left of the entrance towards the "big gallery" there is a poorly illuminated display case with medical instruments—knives, tweezers, tongs.

Over 6,000 artifacts of all types are today displayed in the largest museum of Egyptian art treasures in the world. For systematic construction we thank the French archaeologist Auguste Mariette-Pascha (1821–1881). In the year 1850, as an employee of the Louvre sent to Egypt, he realized success in digging—particularly in Memphis and Abydos. Under his direction on orders from the Khedive, the museum that preceded the present one was founded. After Mariette came his compatriot, Gaston Camille Maspero (1846–1916). The museum has been managed by Egyptian scientists since 1952. Aside from the gigantic exhibits that are organized for visitors, there are vaults and chambers filled with treasures that are intended only for research, which are continually increased by ongoing excavations.

This statue of Iwty is from the Eighteenth or Nineteenth Dynasty. It carried the titles "Chief Physician of the Two Lands" (ie, Upper and Lower Egypt) and "Royal Scribe." In the 3,000 years from Pharaohs Mena to the Ptolemy, Egyptian physicians were viewed so highly that many foreign princes only wanted one gift from the pharaoh: a doctor from the Nile. Homer wrote, "The Egyptians leave the whole world behind in medical knowledge." The physicians were high in the favor of the kings, and their titles are exalted expressions such as "Chief of all court physicians," "Eye physician of the palace," "Physician of the body, who knows the inner juices," "Priest of Aton who in the palace goes and comes and has admission to the king." But the nobles also had their "body physicians," who were employed permanently. In addition, many physicians practiced under orders of the pharaoh in the enormous worker groups: in the Sinai, in copper and turquoise mines, at the temples, in streets, and naturally at pyramid constructions. How these physicians were paid we do not know precisely. Court

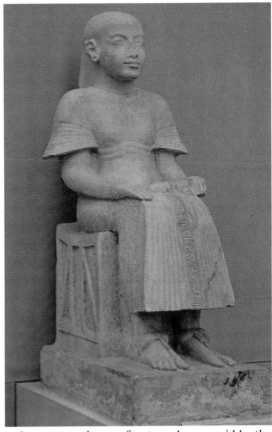

physicians had all the advantages as did those who went to the war fronts and were paid by the pharaoh. General physicians who went into the land were paid with natural products, a gold ring or bracelet—according to conditions. *Dutch Museum, Leiden.*

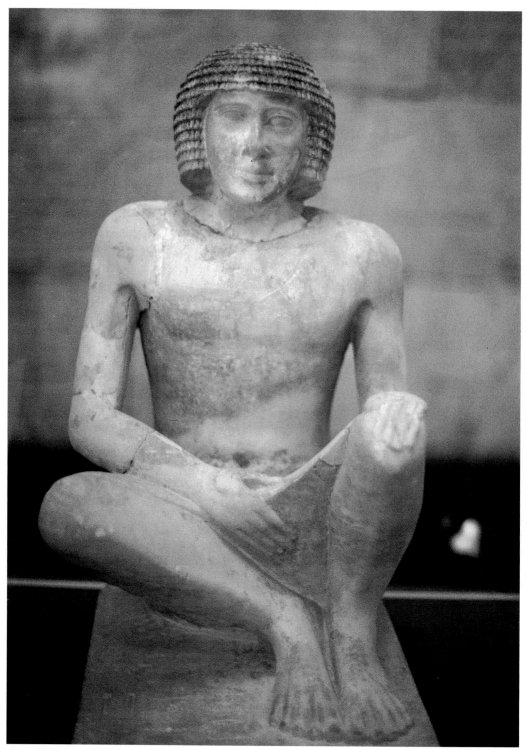

One of the most attractive statues in the museum of Cairo and very unusual artistically because of the position of the legs. Ne-Ankh-Re, chief physician in Giza, at the time of the Eleventh Dynasty. *Egyptian Museum, Cairo.*

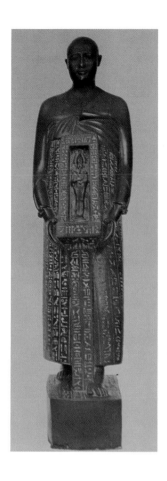

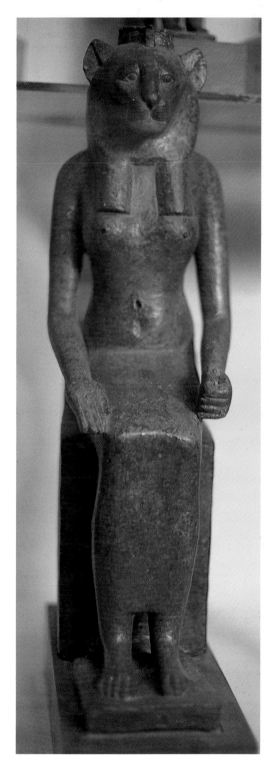

(Above) This is the man who was ordered by King Darius to start the physician's school: Uza-hor-resinet *(wdȝ-ḥ-rśnt·)* of the Twenty-seventh Dynasty. Nevertheless, the statue was found without a head, and another from the same era was placed on the body. The inscription on the body ("Chief of the physicians and royal scribe, friend of the sun, closest to the mother of the gods, Neith, and the goddess of Sais, carrier of the royal seal and his friend, chief of the scribes of the big hall, and of the palace, navigator of the King") is important for science. *Vatican, Rome.*

(Right) Sekhmet, the lion-headed healing goddess who nevertheless was also blamed for many diseases. *Egyptian Museum, Cairo.*

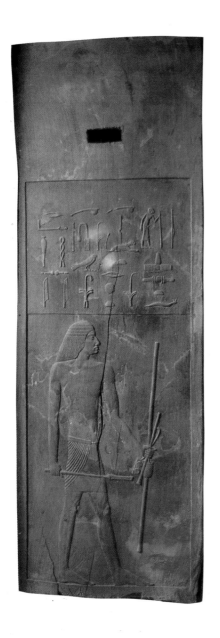
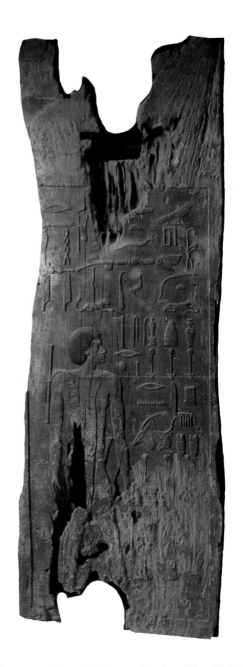

Egyptian scientists are certain that this was the first physician of history: Hesire *(Hsj R')*. He lived at the time of Pharaoh Djoser and seems to have accumulated respectable riches. In Saqqara, Mariette found his tomb—forty-three meters long and over five meters high. It had obviously been robbed several times by tomb robbers. Nearby, the archaeologists found remarkable wall paintings that were not yet usual in the Third Dynasty and six wooden doors with representations of Hesi Re and his profession. The sixth was ruined. These panels are in Cairo today, three are in the large lower hall of the museum and can be seen in the part of the "Old Kingdom." This small alabaster speaks of his name. The inscriptions *(right)* point out Hesi Re as chief physician, Chief of the dentists, architect, scribe, and priest. *Egyptian Museum, Cairo.*

Imhotep
The Doctor
Who Became a God

*So that you know: I was most worried with
my court, because the Nile did not come
in seven years and the entire country was
in great need. Then I turned my heart to
the front; and I asked the wise Imhotep for
advice, where the birthplace of the Nile
is found and who would be the god that
lived there. Upon this Imhotep answered,
"I have to go to the house of books and
look up in the holy books." He returned
soon and revealed wonders to me,
to which no king has ever been shown
the way since the beginning of time . . . .*

Inscription of the "Stele of Famine with the Edict
of Djoser to the Prince of Elephantine" (2780 BC)

More than 100 ancient
Egyptian physicians are known to us
by name; others disappeared in the
duration of time in the "drawers" of
history. For every name that we know
there are probably 1,000 unknown
ones, at least according to the "fathers
of history": Diodorus Siculus, Herodotus of Halikarnassos, and Homer.
They probably wondered, above all,
about the significant level of speciali-
zation that had already been attained
in "the most ancient times." These
knowledge-thirsty "reporters" of ancient times carried the writings
(which we could not read for so long)
to Hellas and ladled information from
these ancient sources of knowledge.
They did not recognize a western
world without Egypt, knowing well

also, that the cradle of Mediterranean culture lies in the Nile. At the time when the oak woods of central Europe were still healthy, sick people died "because of the will of Odin."

Ranking of specialists was as follows: eye doctors were most distinguished, then those doctors who dealt with the head, and in "third place" were dentists. Hesire, who is counted as one of the first physicians of the world, was called about 4,600 years ago, "head of the dentists." At about the same time, the doctor Imhotep ("he who gives contentment") also practiced. He was incomparable to all ancient Egyptian doctors, a truly large and impressive man. He was called to the court of Pharaoh Khasekhem, who had heard about his medical knowledge which had at that time—even without mass media—spread quickly. Numerous legends are attributed to Imhotep from this time on.

It was said that Imhotep came to the Upper Egyptian capital in order to save the life of the great queen. After the birth of prince Djoser, the pharaoh's wife suffered a tear of the perineum. With quick movements, Imhotep bandaged the hemorrhaging and sewed the wound, despite the protestations of the pharaoh's wife and the three midwives. The veterinarian and art reporter, Pierre Montlauer of Toulouse, wrote in his book about Imhotep, "When he was finished, he turned to the speechless women and said, 'on these wounds, compresses of fresh meat must be applied and new ones must be reapplied five times daily. After this, the patient should drink milk mixed with beef gall bladder....'"

The pharaoh's wife survived, yet Imhotep's wife was said to have died during the birth of her son at that same time. The queen's nurse took care of the boy and Imhotep locked himself up with the corpse of his beloved wife for forty days, in order to mummify her—the first time in the history of man (see also the chapter "The Trip to the Other Side").

Imhotep committed a part of his life in deep partiality to the prince (later pharaoh) Djoser, the most important pharaoh of the Third Dynasty. He played a leading role at the court, was a vizier to the king as well as head architect, priest, and astrologist. According to the legend, this "Leonardo of ancient Egypt" (he was also an excellent sculptor) ended a seven-year famine by cleverly devising sophisticated irrigation plans, organizing fisheries, and preserving food. Imhotep also worked on a monument for his pharaoh that is as unique as this artist/physician was himself: he built the first pyramid of the world, the step mastaba of Saqqara. It stands only several kilometers away from Cairo at undoubtedly the most attractive archaeological area of Lower Egypt. The open country of Saqqara is 6,000 meters long and 1,500 meters wide. In it, open graves from the First Dynasty were found above the present town of Abusir. The most important were excavated by

W. B. Emery between 1936 and 1956. The cemetery, which belonged to the ancient capital of Memphis, harbors innumerable graves and underground labyrinths, in which thousands upon thousands of mummified animals lie.

Fifteen royal pyramids are known to us, but it can be assumed that others are hidden under the sands of eternity. One of the best known is important archeologically—that of Unias, the last king of the Fifth Dynasty. It lies in the southwest corner of the "Djoser district," far from the step pyramids. The walls of the interior rooms bore a collection of sayings—advice for all types of ailments in the pharaoh's next life. According to Unias, the pyramid texts, in which the burial ceremonies are also described, belong to the "basic provisions" of the graves of the ancient kingdom and have provided information for all researchers.

To return to Pharaoh Djoser and his physician/architect Imhotep, according to legend, he buried his wife in the desert below the Nile delta and swore to erect a large building over the grave one day. In 2630 BC, the step pyramid originated—the first stone construction of its size in the world. The difficulties in working with new materials (until that time and in many cases today, only dried bricks of mud from the Nile are used) are evident from the hesitant construction of the pyramids. The stone giant underwent six changes in building plans before it grew to its full height. Yet from the beginning, the "wonder

doctor" was also lauded as the "discoverer of the art of construction with chiseled stone." It has been proven that Imhotep did manage the building of the pyramids. During the excavation of the entrance in the years 1925–1926, his name was found on the statue of a pharaoh. And in the next dynasty of the god-king, this type of construction became modern. The erection of the "great pyramid" and the grave of the Pharaoh Khufu (Cheops) in Giza (which was "officially" discovered only in the fourteenth century AD) provides us with a great riddle even today, with its mathematic calculations.

By the beginning of the New Kingdom, Imhotep was honored as a half-god. During the ruling time of Amenophis III, the scribes called to him while they poured drink-offerings out of their water bowls, saying, "Water of the water bowls of every scribe at your Ka, O Imhotep." He was probably already lauded as a healing god at the time of the pyramid-builder Mycerinos in the Fourth Dynasty. The Greeks later saw him as an equal to Asklepios.

Still standing is a list of holy doctors on which Imhotep is cited, along with Amenophis—Hapus' son (under Amenophis III, high ranking military doctor and architect)—and Antinous, who drowned in the Nile and was eaten by crocodiles. Imhotep was favored by King Hadrian, and in Rome, the king had a monument erected to Imhotep. Engraved on one obelisk were the words: "He hears the plea of him who calls him. He lets the needy become well ...."

There were as few female doctor-gods in ancient Egyptian mythology as there were earthly ones. In later times, the Goddess Isis was known to have founded many medications and to be "experienced in healing," which she taught her son Horus. "The magician's mother is the protectress of his limbs and the magician of Horus makes the suffering ones well!"

Ancient Egyptian doctors assumed that, every now and then, their gods also needed medical assistance, hence it was believed that medicine was practiced even into eternity. Those who did this were Amun of Thebes ("who dissolves evil and removes sorrow, the doctor who makes the eye well ... who opens the eyes ...), Thoth ("the doctor of the Horus-eye"), Min, god of Koptos ("the good doctor of he who trusts him") and Horus, as the "head physician in the house of Re." According to legend, Horus himself needed help as he fought to be the heir to Osiris' throne. In the battle, Horus pulled Seth's testicles off, who then revenged himself by striking out one of Horus' eyes. According to legend: "Hathor found Horus as he lay in the desert mountains and cried. She milked a gazelle and said to Horus: open your eye so that I can pour in milk. He opened his eye and she poured milk into it. She put milk into the right one and the left one. She said: open the eye! She looked at him and found him well ...."

Otherwise, an ill god did the same thing as a simple person did: he went to bed! "Here Re says: put him into his bed, may he get well ...."

Disease and Deformity

Obesity, Hunchbacks, and Dwarfs

Do not laugh at a blind one and do
not mock a dwarf.
Do not harm a dumb one and do not
mock a man who is in the hand of
God, and do not be wrathful to him
when he falls.

(Amenemope, 1200 BC)

As we would say today, fat people in ancient Egypt were "out." The ideal woman was slim and willowy and enchanting to look at in her translucent, tightly fitting dress. The man at her side wore, over his small hips, a pleated skirt and had broad shoulders. Obesity was mocked and even caricatured in all epochs by artists. An unusually realistic statue from the Twenty-fifth Dynasty stands in the Egyptian Museum in Cairo. It is of a man with hanging breasts and wobbling stomach at "Harwa," a man of uncertain origin who nevertheless became steward to Queen Amenardeis; at that time, stewardship was a powerful position in the land by the Nile. In addition, he had the title of signet bearer of the king of Lower Egypt and single companion and true truster of God, although he never belonged to the priesthood, because they did not want to have anything to do with a man of Harwa's type. This man's close relationship to the queen, his assignment as head supervisor of the harems, and his significant, although frowned upon, image indicate that he was an eunuch, although there are no real clues.

A rich and respected Egyptian did not want to appear as a fat man to Osiris in his afterlife. Many pictures in the graves are "improved" for this reason. In the mastaba of the Sabu, one sees at the entrance an image of a heavy man. This is probably how Sabu looked originally. However, the farther one ventures into the room of his "eternal life," the more small-hipped and broad-shouldered he becomes.

There are other depictions in the graves of Saqqara, namely a magnificent collection of men with umbilical or scrotal hernia and genital "hypertrophy" (changes in cell or tissue). These depictions are similar to "Egyptian splenomegaly," or infectious swelling caused by many diseases, with hyperfunction a result of multiplied, deteriorating blood cells, different liver diseases, especially thesaurismosis, blood diseases, and obstruction of the liver and spleen circulation. These depictions may relate to an illness that is often described with the word *"âaâ"* in medical books.

Hunchbacks and dwarfs

Dwarfs were highly valued people among the ancient Egyptians. Dwarfs were chosen to look after the wardrobe and the jewelry of the kings and noble men, because if they pinched and ran with the jewels that were entrusted to them, they could be more easily traced than normal-sized men. In addition, the palace dwarfs were allowed to supervise the queen's castle animals. Finally, thanks to their talent on small legs, they were also popular dancers.

In the Egyptian Museum in Cairo there is the statue of a man, about twenty centimeters high, with a sharp hump. Scientists have taken this as an indication that bone tuberculosis was present in ancient Egypt. They also know that the clubbed feet of Menna (a farm inspector) or the poliomyelitis of Pharaoh Siptah are traced back. However, it is not certain whether the long fingers and toes of the priest Meren-Ra-nefer (Sixth Dynasty) point to an inherited heart disease.

An object of study for many medical-historians is Pharaoh Amenhotep IV, who called himself Akhenaten during his reign ("first prophet of Re-Harakhty, who is pleased at the horizon in the name of Schu, who is Aten). The complicated name is the beginning of the atonic religion. According to the opinion of the pharaohs, Re-Harakhty continually created his life anew, and "Schu" is interpreted as sunlight in this context. "Aten" is the power that combines everything. Akhenaten was married to a woman of unknown origin, although possibly she was Asian. As she moved into "Thebes with a hundred gateways" with a great entourage and greater dowry, the people gave her the name Nefertiti, "the beauty has arrived." Akhenaten was, next to her, less majestic, even ugly, with his soft figure, feminine breasts, filled-out hips, sunken stomach, and an "egghead." But his smug arrogance must have made an impression on his contemporaries, because they all wanted to look like the "great renewer." Until the mummy of the pharaoh is identified without a doubt, it is left open as to whether the depiction actually corresponds to his appearance, or if it was merely an expression of the new "sun cult," which Akhenaten had imported. Otherwise, the fat stomach and gynecomastism (development of female-like breasts in men) are symbols for "fruitful" characters like Hapi (the master of the floods) or Npri (the master of the wheat).

There are also depictions, not of small funny figures with rolls of fat, but of a more accurate pathologic quality, as in a medical textbook. The best example is Ati, the king of the neighboring country Punt. A relief from the temple of Hatshepsut in Deir el Bahari (named for a Coptic cloister, which was built later) shows the queen as she brings gifts to the pharaoh's wife. She looks terrible: bags of flesh hang from her arms and thighs and only the joints of her hands and ankles are visible. Her disease has been diagnosed as either elephantitis (thick skin resulting from an obstruction of the lymphatic system), as myxoedema (saturation of the subcutaneous tissue with colloid substances as a result of decreased activity or absence of activity of the thyroid gland), or as dystrophia musculorum (chronic degeneration of the skeletal muscles, probably from an inherited disturbance of the enzymatic function). The relief shows that the daughter has the first signs of this disease.

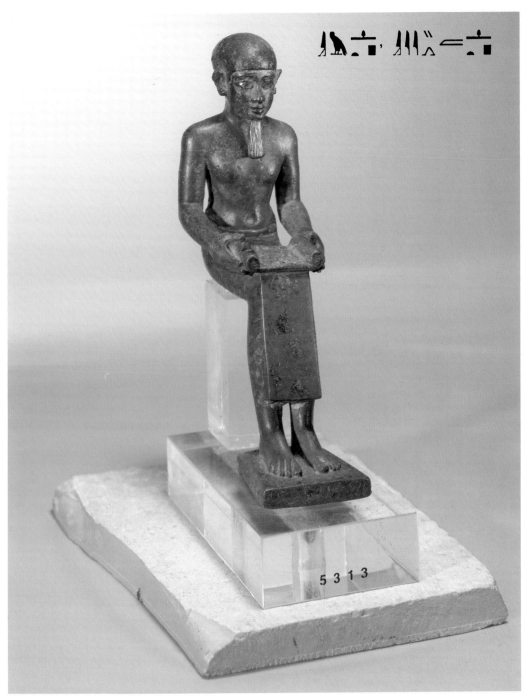

Imhotep. This man was of universal skill: human, but during his lifetime revered as a healing god. He entered history differently from Hesi Re or Irj. As physician of the pharaoh he constructed the first pyramid of the world. He lived at the time of Pharaoh Djoser and is on a Graffitto of the Third Dynasty on the surrounding wall of the pyramid's region referred to as Horus-Sakhmet (early Old Kingdom). *State Collection of Egyptian Art, Munich.*

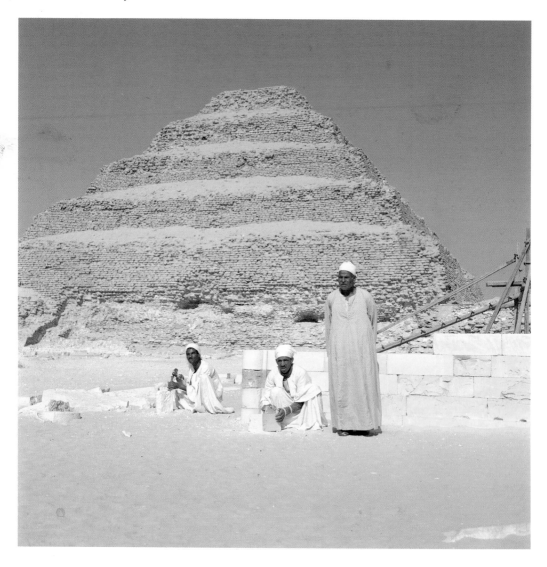

(Above)   This is what Imhotep created, along with many other things. It is the first pyramid of the world, the so-called step mastaba in Saqqara. Many legends discuss its construction. It had been planned as a tomb for Pharaoh Djoser, but is Imhotep's wife under it? Imhotep was already considered the son of the celestial father Ptah in the Old Kingdom. Only in this way could he, as a normal human, be so acquainted with the supernatural. Someone who could do as much as Imhotep had to be associated with the gods. Physician, sculptor, architect, knowledgeable in the writing arts, reading priests—the man knew all. The Greeks "recognized" him later as their healing god "Asklepios." The terrain around the step mastaba is still today one of the most interesting excavation areas of the world.

(Right)   This bust is considered a "master portrait of history." As the fine lady arrived in Thebes—no one knows from where—to become the wife of Akhenaten, the masses were perplexed. "The beautiful arrived" was the saying, which is translated "Nefertiti." *State Museums, Berlin.*

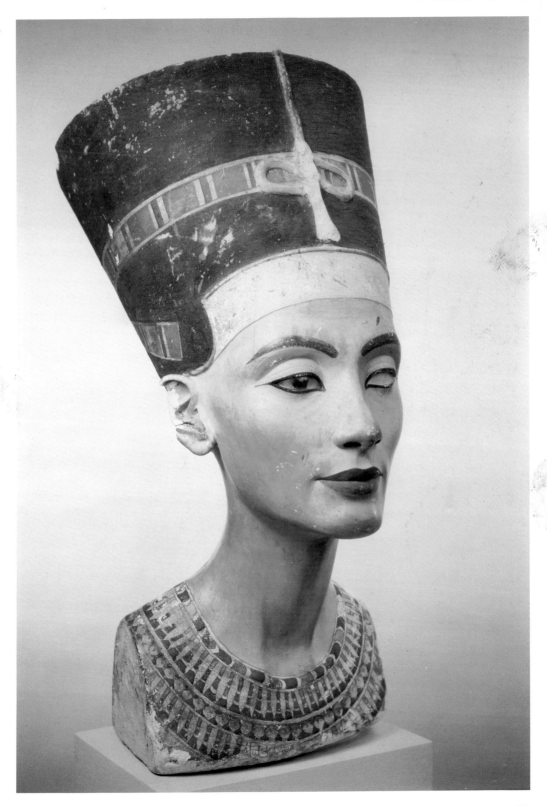

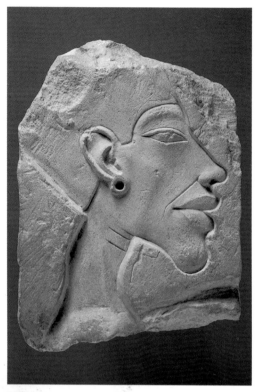

(Left)   One of the most glittering figures of Egyptian history: Pharaoh Amenophis IV from the Eighteenth Dynasty. He was a female-appearing but ascetic-appearing type who wanted to introduce a new religion into Egypt: the sun as the only deity. He had spent his youth in the palace of his father in Malgata on the western shore of Thebes. As king he founded the city "Horizon of the sun shine" (Tell el-Amar-nan or short: Amarna) and called himself "the docile to Aton": Akhenaten. He associated (since he remained without a throne-following) a relative— Smenkhkare— in the government. Since they died one shortly after the other, a solution to the problem had to be found in a hurry since Egypt was sinking into anarchy. The power was turned over to another relative, his name: Tutankhamun, ten years old. He later placed the traditional gods in their old rites and changed his name to Amun. *State Museums, Berlin.*

(Below)   An Amarna relief with the name: Olive branch for Aton. *Schimmel Collection, New York.*

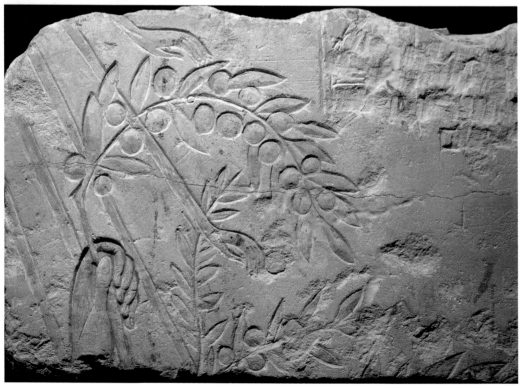

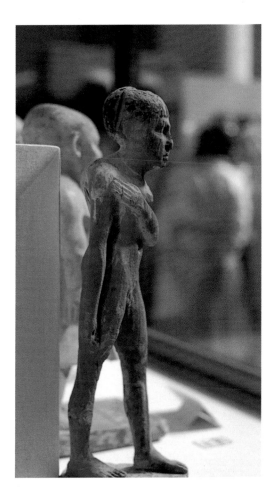

Based on this twenty-centimeter-high sculpture, scientists concluded that tuberculosis of the bone was present in ancient Egypt. Malformations were frequent. The Pharaoh Siptah, for example, lived with club feet, which suggests childhood spinal paralysis. *Egyptian Museum, Cairo.*

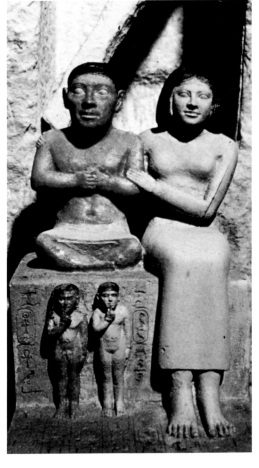

Dwarfs were highly regarded in ancient Egypt. They were in charge of the cloak-room and jewelry of the pharaoh and took care of the domestic animals. They were also valued because of their comical effect as dancers. This plaster sculpture from the Cairo museum shows the dwarf, Seneb, with his totally normal family. *Egyptian Museum, Cairo.*

77

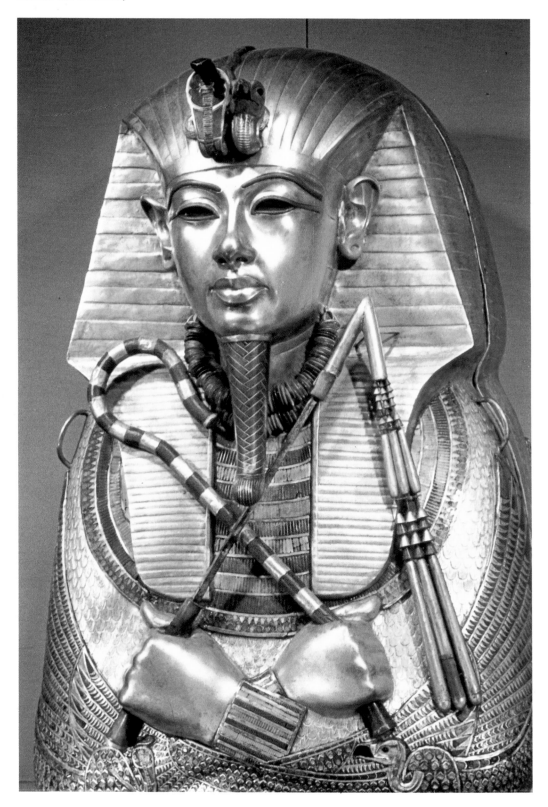

(Left) Detail of the gold coffin from the tomb of Pharaoh Tutankhamun. His corpse was placed in three coffins and four shrines. The head and shoulders were covered with a gold mask. The sarcophagus was in an exact east-west direction and 143 objects had been placed with the mummy for company. The head was covered by a gold-and-precious-stone diadem, with the religious sign of the Upper and Lower Kingdoms. The entrance to the dead young pharaoh's tomb was discovered by Howard Carter in November, 1922. On the pharaoh's throat was a symbolic collar of twenty amulets placed in six rows. On his chest, arms, and fingers were gold jewelry and pearls. His feet were placed in gold sandals. Incredible wealth was found in one of the smallest tombs in the Valley of the Kings. *Egyptian Museum, Cairo.*

(Below) Tutankamun's tomb is not far from Deir el-Bahari, where the temple of Hatshepsut is. It is located on the west side of the Nile, exactly opposite to Karnak, and is impressive because of the majestic rocks behind it. The temple is a gigantic construction of the only female pharaoh that Egypt ever had. Mostly, however, it exposes the in-fighting for power among the members of a family.

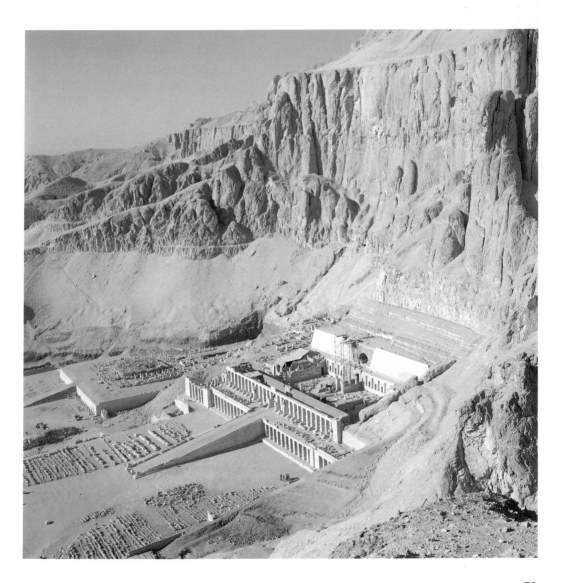

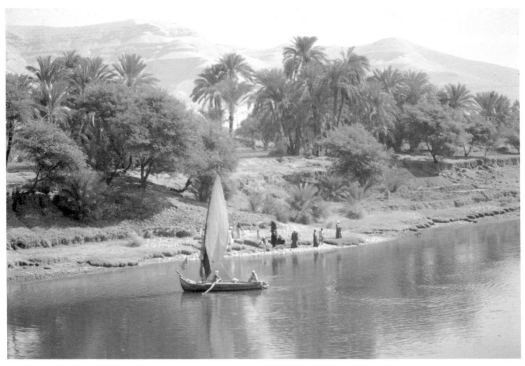

The Nile is 6,500 kilometers long and for centuries it determined the history of the land. Famine years and rich corn, fish blessings, and fruitful mud from middle Africa were brought to the population, as was a very dangerous disease.

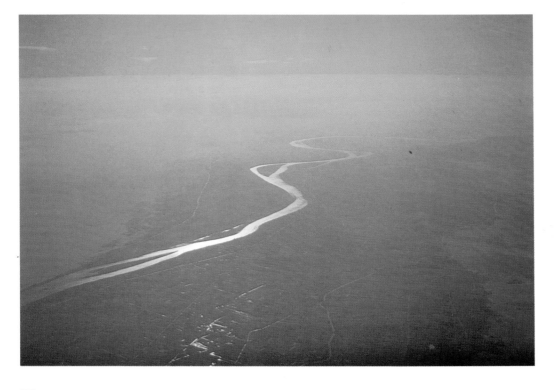

Travels With Hatshepsut

*The body of the human is wider than
a barn and full of answers; choose the
good ones and say them, let the bad ones
be locked in your body.*
(*Teaching of Anii, 1350 BC*)

Here let us briefly allow
ourselves a breather from medicine
and spend some time in the shady
columns of the temple of Deir el
Bahari. During the time when the
beautiful Princess Hatshepsut (of the
Eighteenth Dynasty) had the semi-cir-
cular basin built, she called the place
"Zoser-Zosru," the "Holy of the Holy."
The colossal construction is a must-
see for every tourist caravan that has
earlier sailed in luxury over the Nile
and then been driven into the Valley
of the Kings. One busload chases another through the small streets to the
temple of Hatshepsut. One should
ignore the smiling looks of the taxi
and bus drivers (their greed for tourist
money has robbed them of their last
sparks of common sense) and go over
the mountain on foot. A few steps
away from the left-hand side of Tutankhamun's grave, the path begins.
After a quarter hour of walking
(admittedly, one begins to breathe
heavily), one experiences Egypt in a
way that Hatshepsut loved. The Nile
snakes through the desert, bordered
by narrow strips of green land, until it

reaches the pyramid in the horizon. The Memnon-Colossian (in ancient times they still belonged to the seven wonders of the world) lie clearly visible in the valley underneath and back of the temple of Karnak. This hike is worthwhile!

The Temple of Hatshepsut is interesting for two reasons: for one, there is no building in Egypt whose remains (beautifully restored by a Polish archaeologist) make the power struggle of a family so clearly visible. In the temple inscriptions, everything revolves around the only female pharaoh, "She is like godly breath, her skin is golden and shines like the stars. She is a great wonder. She was singled out to protect Egypt because of her gift, to make men want to be brave. She lives, she is steadfast, she is of good health. She is . . . for always and forever." But even the name of her father Tuthmosis I and her brother Tuthmosis II appear. In addition, Tuthmosis III appears, who married her daughter and after the death of Hatshepsut and his assent to the throne had his aunt's figures and cartouches chiseled out of the reliefs. This action satisfied the hate he had as reigning monarch against the superior "female government" that Hatshepsut had built. (It must be conceded, however, that once he stepped out of the shadow, he became a powerful personality. Under his single government, Egypt became an empire that reached from the Euphrates to the Sudan. In seventeen campaigns, he overthrew the kingdoms of Palas-tine, Phoenix, and North Syria. With energy and political perspicacity, he secured Egypt's supremacy at that time in the world.)

Akhenaten's followers later destroyed much in the gigantic temple; Sethos I and Ramses II restored it again, although the two were vain enough to have everything painted over with their own cartouches. What remains are depictions of dignitaries of Hatshepsut's court, below Senenmut, the architect of the temple, who rose from a small priest-youth to become "royal signet-bearer" and educator of Hatshepsut's children (very possibly his own). He was the great and only love of the queen, who, despite the masculine behavior she had to display during her reign (even wearing a ceremonial beard) she did not want to deny herself.

In 1495 BC, Hatshepsut organized an expedition to the African country Punt (the course of this expedition an artist later chiseled in the south wall of the temple). Such expeditions had, at that time, all kinds of medical reasons. The priests and physicians became dissatisfied with the plants and drugs of their homeland. For example, there was no antimony on the Nile, rather only along the banks of the Sambesi. It is not known where Punt must have been, but the travel route was probably as follows: from the harbor Leukos Limos—or Philoteras—on the Red Sea, the captains with their crews shipped through the Gulf of Aden, past Saba (Yemen today) to the Indian Ocean.

They sailed along the African coast, past the Comoros, and anchored before Zimbabwe, probably Punt at that time.

With astounding wonder the travellers viewed the tropically abundant plant world, which is still today our most important pharmacy (forty percent of all our medicines come from the tropical forests around the equator). In comparison, Egypt's local flora left much to be desired. Amazed, the travellers stepped into the villages of the natives. There were no palaces or brick houses, only small huts that looked like bees' nests standing under trees on posts. The entrance to the huts, as big as a hole, could only be reached on a ladder. This must have seemed astonishingly backwards to an Egyptian whose forefathers had already built pyramids 146 meters high!

The natives living in the huts approached, wearing loincloths, massive jewelry, and dirty hair (this was "shocking" for someone from the Nile: see the chapter on hygiene) braided against their heads. "Truly untouched by every culture," the head of the expedition (in the reliefs of Deir el-Bahari he was called Nehsi) must have uttered, and then the man from thirty-four centuries ago, saw, shuddering, the chief named Perihu coming, leading a donkey by a rope on top of which sat the fat chief's wife, Ati. But the expedition team did not even sail as far as the Mosern. The leader did what a Carthaginian merchant of the fifth century BC, or a captain of the sixteenth or seventeenth century AD did: he opened a market. He traded preserves, daggers, slaughtering axes, and bright trinkets for the treasures of Punt: heaps of incense-resin, ivory, myrrh trees; ebony, gold, and eye jewelry; baboons, long-tailed monkeys, afghans, panther furs; and naturally, even a few slaves.

Different and more dangerous expeditions were made into the land. Through deserts and swamps, steppes and jungles, the Egyptians tried to force their way into inner Africa. Death has always been a reliable companion on the road to important medicines. They searched for the "salt of the desert," yellow ochre and malachite, acacia, and Ami-Majos—a root that, when chewed, protects against the sun. Current research has found a material in this root that supports the building of pigment in the skin and causes artificial tanning. Medicine has benefitted from valuable minerals and drugs from the south of Africa, the land of Kusch (Nubia, Ethiopia), and this is covered in more detail in the chapter "Remedies."

Love, Lust, and Birth

I will lie down in my house,
I will lie ill, something will happen to me,
And the neighbors will visit me.
My sister will come too,
And my sister will shame all,
Yes, she will shame the physicians
Because my sister knows my disease.
(Love song dating from the New Kingdom)

In ancient Egypt girls usually married at the age of twelve or thirteen years, men at age fifteen. Marriages between brothers and sisters were common, especially in the ruling houses. This is because it was important to keep a god's blood pure, and the pharaohs were descendents of the gods. Also, mythology held that the goddess Isis had married her brother, Osiris, and Nephthys married her brother Seth. Eventually, people started imitating this practice more often; in the second century AD, two thirds of the marriages in the city of Arsinoe were brother-sister marriages. The Greeks observed this with great surprise.

As will be discussed further when examining mummies, many scientists are of the opinion that incest is the reason for the hereditary diseases of generations of pharaohs. This was contradicted in a study by Marc Armand Ruffer in 1919. He was of the opinion that brother-sister marriages did not have an adverse genetic effect. The Eighteenth Dynasty, in which incest was common, brought nine great personalities to history. And, of the fourteen Ptolemy kings, the first four were not married to blood relatives yet the other ten were as normal as they were. In total, they lived to an average age of sixty-four years (save for one assassination).

Sex life in ancient Egypt, contrary to the views of Christianity, was not considered a sin. It was only forbidden to take one's pleasure in the temple, or to enter the temple after sex and without cleansing. Among common people, a single marriage was the rule, but men—who could afford to—had harems, and slave girls were, of course, available to the men. Slaves were also the inhabitants of the many brothels spread around the country, provided the slaves were not being used by the owners. So they were able to earn some money and basically have fun with it.

Herodotus tells in his history that men would only give a dead wife to the embalmer after several days had passed because they were afraid the embalmer would "take advantage" of the women. He also noted—a fact completely unbelievable for a Greek—that Pharaoh Rampisint sent his own daughter to the bordello as a means of obtaining information on the thoughts of the populace. Therefore, it is perhaps not surprising that Ramses II slept with each of his fifty daughters. Not only people and kings took part in this sinful amusement, but the gods did as well. The god of fruitfulness, Min, is always represented with an erect penis. And the bad mood of the sun god, Re, improved only on a day when the sky goddess Hathor removed her clothes.

Fear of having too many children was unknown because children were cheap labor and the death rate was quite high. Herodotus wrote that a woman needed to get pregnant twelve times in order to have at least two children survive. According to his statistics, she would have had eight miscarriages, and of four children, two would die in the first three years. Pharaoh Ramses II—energetic in all respects—had 170 children in the course of his life; Baba (an official of the Middle Kingdom) had sixty. Despite such tendencies of prolific reproduction, contraceptive measures were known. One recipe states that one should "finely grind acacia points with dates and honey, apply on a tampon, and place deep in the womb." Since then it has been discovered that acacia points contain a type of rubber that on solution produces lactic acid. Lactic acid is also present in current contraceptives.

Prostitution (which also occurred among men) was in all senses acceptable, since a sense of shame as we know it did not exist. Special provocative outfits would have been unnecessary, but even to an ancient Egyptian an excitingly covered woman was more interesting than a naked one. Therefore, the tight, slightly transparent dresses were made of linen (silk was unknown). Working women, handmaids, and dancers, like men, wore only a loincloth or a belt which was knotted in the front. Only during the New Kingdom did the loincloth become, after being very carefully worked, a skirt. And on festive occasions a wig was also worn. The wig, however, was also used as an erotic signal. There is a story dating to the New Kingdom of a woman who blamed her brother-in-law for wanting to seduce her. Her proof was in his words, "Come, we shall have fun and sleep together. Put on your wig."

Although pornographic material was found in many tombs (so that the dead should have fun on their way to eternity) there is nothing about sex in the old writings, except in poetic form:

Seven days were it yesterday that I have not seen my beloved. A suffering penetrated me, and I became heavy in my body, and I did not know further. When the chief physicians came, my heart was not refreshed from their medicines. The priest did not bring help; my suffering could not be judged. [However] he told me: there she is! He kept me alive. Her name is what has kept me erect, the coming and going of her boat is what keeps my heart alive. More important than all medicines is my beloved, more important than a whole book of recipes.

Ptahotep recommends the following in his "Wisdoms": "When you are respected, establish a household and love your wife at home as is proper. Fill her womb and cover her back. The medicine for her limbs is soap oil. Delight her heart as long as she lives. She is good soil for her master."

In regard to intercourse there is usually talk of pregnancy, "... he slept with his wife at night: she conceived and became pregnant. He recognized her in the recognition of a man. She became pregnant in the night with a small boy ...."

In legend there is description of the creation of the future Pharaoh Hatshepsut. According to the legend, the god Amun was Hatshepsut's father, not Pharaoh Tuthmosis I, although her mother was the pharaoh's wife, Ahmes. Amun discovered that "the queen, Ahmes, is a virgin, prettier than any other woman." He "made his appearance to be like that of King Tuthmosis" and found the queen as "she rested in bed, in the beauty of her palace. She awoke with the perfume of the god. She smiled at the appearance of his majesty. He advanced at her. He gave her his heart. He allowed her to see him in the real appearance of the god, after having posed to her, and she was happy with his beauty. His love penetrated her body...." There are gaps in the text, "he had all he wanted in her... after the majesty of the god did all he wanted with her..." said the queen, "... my master! How big is your force. It is marvelous to see you from the front. You have united my majesty with your marvelous force. Your fragrance melts my whole body." Amun then tells her about the "daughter that I placed in your stomach." As a god he would know that he had produced the one who later would become the female Pharaoh Hatshepsut. (Translation is from K. Sethe, "Origin of the Eighteenth Dynasty I," Leipzig, Germany: Engelmann, 1914. Grapow has given the wording more precisely.)

There are no descriptions in the usual texts of how one discovered pregnancy and how it developed. The duration was calculated as in the present day as nine months, in contrast to the Hebrews and Greeks, according to whose calendar it was ten months. Labor pains, however, are described, "... as the woman, who is pregnant with three children ... suffered and it became painful, that she would deliver ... the divine father sent four female midwives ...."

At delivery only female helpers were present, not physicians. The god Khnum, who gave health to the newborn according to legend, only did so after birth. Queen Ahmes prayed to Amun as she was in labor, "Speed up as the northwinds. The pregnancy has taken its time, it is painful, the time has come ...." The peasant woman, when her time of delivery approached, called to her side two women, either from her household or neighbors who could help her. She would place two small statues, representations of Taweret and Bes, as not to be an "easy prey" for bad spirits.

Taweret was the protective patroness of all pregnant women and was represented as a hippopotamus standing on its hind legs. She had once delivered the Earth, and her image was carved in amulets. In Berlin there are large statues of Tawaret. In two the dresses can be removed, and in the third there are holes in the breasts. These statues were probably filled with milk that dropped from the new mother's breasts, perhaps in the hopes that her milk supply should not dry up.

As for Bes, he is a very ugly gnome with a large stomach and an animal face. He was usually represented in a panther skin with hanging claws and carried a wild headdress. His ugliness was his power since it scared all that was bad. His representation has been found on mirror handles, perhaps so that a woman could avoid irritating the gods when she regarded herself pleasantly or when she painted herself.

Women delivered their babies while on their haunches. Either the pregnant woman kneeled or sat on her heels, or a "delivery seat" was constructed with bricks so that the child had more space. Often, hot water was placed under the seat so that the vapors would make delivery easier. At the same time, "delivery sayings" were repeated, such as the one that asked Amun to "make the heart of the deliverer strong, and keep alive the one that is coming."

In the northern corridor of the temple of Kom Ombo (located about half an hour from Asswan, directly on the Nile highway) there is a beautiful representation chiseled in the wall showing how Isis brought a child into the world in this manner. Next to it is the only representation of surgical instruments (see photograph on page 58) that have been found in Egypt.

"Intoxicating resources" that were used by women during delivery is demonstrated in a statement found in the delivery temple of Edfu, "Happy is the face of the delivering person when she is drunk in response to the jug of the beer goddess ...."

Delivery is described in a legend in the Papyrus Westcar. A pregnant priestess is delivered with the help of the goddesses Isis, Nephthys, and Heket (in the form of a frog). "They appeared to the woman. They closed the room. Isis placed herself in front of her, Nephthys in the back. Heket made the delivery fast. The child slid in her hands as a child of a poker. She washed it, and cut the umbilicus off.... The priestess 'cleaned' herself with a cleaning of

fourteen days." Although we do not know exactly what this final statement means, it does bring to mind the "confinement" of our days. Whether the newborn would survive was tested in the following manner: "Dissolve a crumb of the placenta in milk and give it to him for three days ... if he vomits it, he will die ...."

For three years the baby was fed mother's milk or the milk of a wet nurse ("as you were born after your months, her breast was in your mouth for three years ..."). Special medicines were used to increase milk production.

Finally, on the topic of childbearing, in a complaint letter against "many persons," we read of "death from the removal of a pregnancy." A man is blamed for influencing the "removal in delivering a woman." It seems that abortion was practiced.

Practical Therapeutics

"First the teeth, then the eyes"

Become an expert in your eyes, take care that another one does not become more knowledgeable.
(Lesson of Djedefhor, circa 2650 BC)

The teeth

All texts available to us make clear the high position of dental medicine among the medical arts. Marc Armand Ruffer together with Elliott Smith studied many mummy skulls dating from the time of the first dynasties to Roman days and found alveolar abscesses, dental caries, and tartar formation. These problems were probably the result of deficient nutrition (more on this later) of the poorer segments of the population. According to the studies of the pathologist (Ruffer), a decisive factor for many was flour, which often contained remnants of the milling stone.

The Papyrus Ebers (nos. 554 and 746) describes inflammation of the teeth and gingiva, and in no. 739 we find fragments of a dental monograph titled "The Beginning of Remedies for Stronger Teeth." Carious teeth were treated with a mixture of ocher, flour, spelt, and honey; fillings were also made with a combination of malachite and resin.

Surgical interventions have not been found in texts, although archaeological finds show technical attempts. In the Harvard University Museum there is a mandible from the Fourth Dynasty (around 2600 BC) that shows traces of a drill. It is thought that drainage of abscesses was created by the use of heated drills.

In the shaft of a mastaba in Giza, two teeth were found in 1929 that were artfully fixed with a gold wire—the first prosthesis perhaps? Artificial teeth in the jaws of mummies were also found by researchers.

An interesting "dental story" has been left to us by Ebers in his book *An Egyptian King's Daughter*. It is briefly extracted:

... the boor Aristomachus, however, I must thank. He has considerably furthered the aim of my trip to Egypt. I came here to have a bad tooth removed by an Egyptian dentist who is able to remove diseased teeth without much pain. Aristomachus removed the damaged part of my dentition with his punch and in this manner avoided for me the operation I was so fearful of. As I came back to my senses, I found three teeth that had been knocked out of my mouth: one diseased tooth, and two good ones in which one could see that they might have given me trouble in the future....

The eyes

The prince's daughter wore a heavy, black wig in which two rows of lotus blossoms were arranged artfully. On her neck a chain shone in the form of a fan, made of gold and ceramic beads with turquoise color fringes. The cloth of white linen, which covered her body tightly from the breast to the hips to the ankles, allowed the complete figure to be imagined. "You will do everything to let me see again, won't you physician?" She took a step forward, without help, in her blindness.

"First I want to examine my patient," he said. "I do not need soldiers for that." "Go away," ordered the prince to his guards. The physician took a pouch with herbs from the basket which he carried with him and ordered that hot water be brought. "Sit down," he said. "I will bring you to the seat, and then you can tell me of your eye pain. First, however, I will raise your lids and inflict pain."

She said, "I know that it hurts, I already tried it myself, but the sun blinded me again."

"So the vision has been maintained!"

Tears mixed with pus fell from her eyes. "Three days ago," she said, "it started as I was painting myself."

"Now courage. At the end of the pain is the cure."

This scene of eye treatment was supposed to have happened when the physician Imhotep was taken to the daughter of a prince who had changed her eye makeup. The inflammation involved ingrown eyelashes. The physician pulled with the tweezers, cleaned, massaged with a cream of frankincense and galenicals. Finally he placed on the handsome lady a wet dressing over the eyes....

Again, it is Herodotus who reports on the high respect that ancient Egyptians had for eye doctors. The Persian king Cyros (died in 529 BC) wanted nothing with greater longing from Pharaoh Amasis of Egypt than the best eye physician as medical counselor.

From an anatomical point of view, the Egyptians knew only the external part of the eye. They differentiated "roots" (the lateral muscles of the eye bulb), eyelashes, and lids as well as the pupil and the white of the eye. Sometimes they also distinguished between pupil and iris (elsewhere we have already discussed the relationship between the ear and the eye through the temple and the four vessels.) Nevertheless, they distinguished between an "external" and an "internal" eye treatment. Considered incurable, of course, was total blindness because it was a "punishment of the gods." Then there were the eye diseases as a consequence of damage to the organ or as part of the aging process, and there was acute injury (for example, injury that took place during work, in stone cutting or construction at the mountains). These "external" eye injuries were treated with tinctures that the physician placed on the eye with a vulture quill (the precursor of our pipette). Such a treatment is well represented by the artists who decorated the tomb of

Pharaoh Ipy. For instance, a physician takes care of a worker who has a splinter in his eye from working on Ipy's sarcophagus (nearby, in the same drawing, another physician settles the shoulder of another worker who is lying down in the same way as is described in the Papyrus Smith).

From then until today, eye diseases have been more frequent in Egypt than in other lands, which may be due to the Nile and the unusual climatic changes that occur during the year. A list of the sufferings from which the ancient Egyptians were afflicted includes: varied types of inflammations, leukomas (white opacification of the cornea), morbid tearing, night blindness, ulcers of the cornea, green and gray cataracts, chalazia (inflammation of the meibomian glands, which requires surgery), ectropion (inversion of the eyelids), and strabismus (squint) in all forms.

The worst, however, was (and still is) trachoma, or "corneal illness." It is contagious, causes fifty percent of all blindness, and is also known as "Egyptian eye disease." Trachoma is an infection of the conjunctiva that is endemic in tropical lands, can become epidemic, and must be reported. The causative agent is the bacteria *Chlamydia trachomatis*, which forms many follicles (blisters) on the surface of the conjunctiva. They cause a chronic conjunctival inflammation and finally total blindness. Trachoma is the major cause of blindness in the world with about half a billion people afflicted. This disease, transmitted by flies, was treated by eye specialists with a mixture of sodium carbonate, black mascara, and red ocher.

Against blindness, the Papyrus Ebers no. 356 recommends: "Mix both eyes of a pig, ground with black mascara, red ocher, and honey, place in the ear of the patient." Night blindness should be cured by eating cow's liver (vitamin A!) (Papyrus Ebers no. 351).

Inflammation of the edge of the lid was treated with a mixture of acacia, green eye mascara, and bitter apple. To treat eyelashes that grew inward and damaged the cornea, Egyptian eye physicians—after having removed the offending eyelashes—would coat the area with resin mixed with bat and lizard blood.

Whether gray cataracts were treated we cannot be sure of—there is no discussion of it in the papyri. However, the Babylonians and Assyrians left the information that cataracts could be treated if one removed from the vision area the nontransparent part of the lens inside the eye (using a needle). The Egyptians probably knew this too. The Greco-Roman physician Galen (AD 129–199) told his Emperor Marcus Aurelius (de partibus art. med. lib.) that cataract operations were performed in Alexandria.

Mascara of different compositions was used for medicinal as well as cosmetic purposes. There was a mascara for each time of the year, and it seems that the different compositions had antiseptic effects. The physicians' knowledge of this field is remarkable.

Black mascara that was found on the mummies at Achmim was made from a mixture of lead sulfate and coal. The Egyptians only knew of pure lead. They probably transformed lead flakes by heating them in air, which they then dissolved with vinegar, and by the addition of alumina they formed lead. By heating this product with coal, they made black mascara.

Examination of a paste from the British Museum showed that it was composed of verdigris and resin. Other samples usually had lead oxide or antimony oxide—two ores that were never available in Egypt (perhaps they were obtained from the expedition of Hatshepsut).

The physician Hugo Magnus also examined the mascara at the turn of the century. He found pyrolusite, pulverized copper oxide that became incandescent with carbonate, iron oxide, and a brown mascara with a high component of iron oxide. In addition, the Egyptians used as eye medicine a salve made with honey with *Ricinus* (it is not only a purgative, it also heals wounds), and wood powder of mountain ash, which absorbed inflammatory exudates. (Magnus was of the opinion that artificial eyes were also used. He based that in part on a statement from the Talmud: "It is said for a maiden of the Nile that one made her an artificial tooth and an artificial eye.")

Even in our century, treatment with copper pins (and if this could not be tolerated, alum pins) was recommended in home medicine, and it is still common to use bandages with boric acid or clay and vinegar.

For packaging of mascara, finger-thick stalks or dicotyledon leaves were used, and for storage, alabaster or clay containers. Queens carried on trips (as is also the custom today) a mascara case, and among the treasures of the tomb of Tutankhamun, Howard Carter found a mascara palette for six colors.

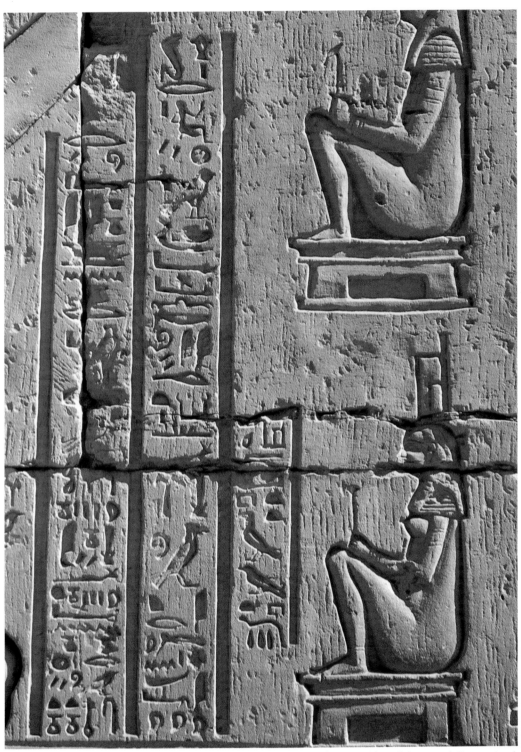

A picture that has not been seen before: a representation of the goddess Isis on a delivery stool. In ancient Egypt women brought children into the world while in a crouching position. *Temple of Com Ombo.*

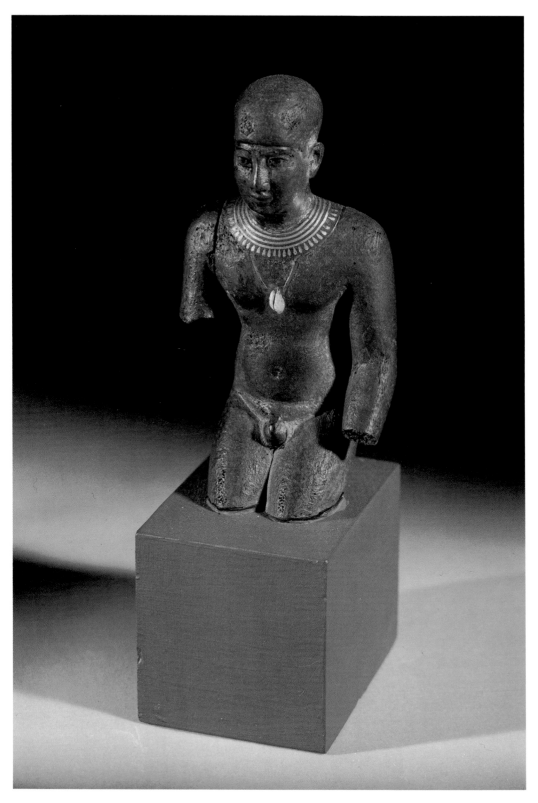

(Left) This nine-centimeter-tall bronze statue is from the fourth century BC and shows Harpokrates, the son of Isis and Osiris. *Schimmel Collection, New York.*

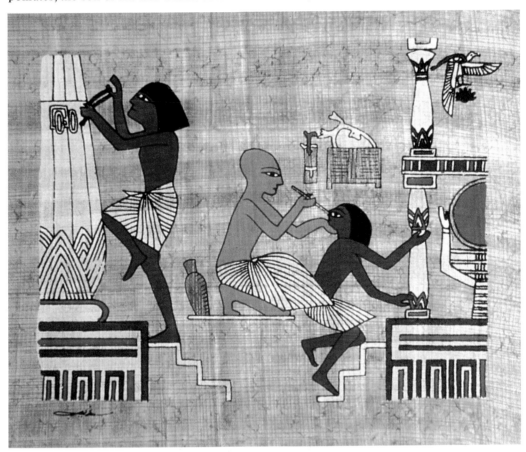

(Above) This (new) papyrus from an old wall painting shows the treatment of a patient by an eye physician. The patient is a stone cutter who received a splinter in the eye while working. The Greek historian Herodotus tells of the high level of Egyptian eye physicians and of their high regard in his *Histories.* Therefore, the Persian king Cyrus (died 529 BC) requested from Pharaoh Amasis nothing more important than the best eye physician of Egypt as a medical consultant.

(Right) Eye diseases are often seen in Egypt today. On expeditions, remedies for their treatment were sought which were then placed in expensive containers. *Egyptian Museum, Cairo.*

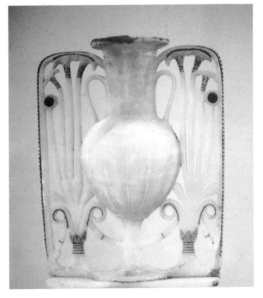

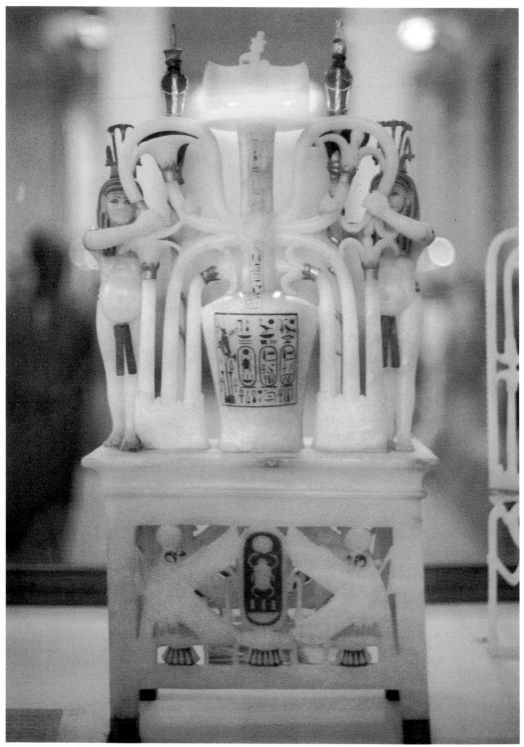

A container for ointments from the tomb chamber of Tutankhamun. Alabaster with gold and ivory. Gods with lotus and papyrus hold thin columns with the king's uraeus (serpent). *Egyptian Museum, Cairo.*

Magical-Religious Treatments

*"They have given me their protection ...
I am one, from whom God wants, that he
keeps me alive."*
(Papyrus Ebers)

It is Cairo in the heat of early summer. A tiny elevator, in which instead of three, seven people sweat, brings us to the fourth floor of the "Department of Antiquities." There, Dr Ali Hassan stands guard behind a busy outer office of Egypt's older treasures. Dr Hassan, a doctoral graduate of Göttingen in archaeology and former director of the Cairo Museum, is a specialist for archaeology and religion and is more knowledgeable than any other regarding medicine and magic. Between the hum of the ventilator and the uninterrupted ringing of the telephone, he says, "Magic and medicine and the religious motive behind the healing of the ill are hard to separate. Magic treatments still live today; the Egyptians of our day do many things exactly as they did thousands of years ago. In ancient Egypt, religion and magic carried the same weight; the patient trusted the word of the priest as much as the knowledge of his physician. And naturally, one tried to bring in the role of the gods through magic. Especially for incurable illnesses, such as cancer."

For Dr Hassan and many other scientists, it is clear that the ancient Egyptians knew about cancer. We know the diagnosis for a woman's disease from the Papyrus Kahun (no. 2) (unfortunately, the text allows for several interpretations), that is as follows: "Treatment for a woman whose ḥm·t (uterus) became ill . . . ." F. L. Griffith, the first to work on the text, wrote, "This may be cancer (carcinoma uteri) which is characterized by a peculiar smell" (in Papyrus Kahun it was noted that the woman emitted "an odor that smelled like roast meat"). Then there is the opposing opinion of the German K. Sudhoff in a presentation in 1933 on "Cancerous Growths in the Ancient Egyptian Papyri," which H. E. Sigerist summarized in 1951 in the *History of Medicine,* "Sudhoff examined all passages which might refer to cancer and came to the conclusion that it was impossible to tell from extant literature whether the Egyptians knew of cancer."

We go now from Cairo into the Bavarian city of Regensburg. There, Dr Christa Habrich (with Drs Dietrich Wildung, Kamal Sabri Kolta, and Sylvia Schoske) prepared in 1985 an exhibit in the German Medical History Museum, "Medicine in Ancient Egypt." In an accompanying text, the exhibitors noted:

The prominent direction of religious thinking in ancient Egypt is the belief of the existence of an unlimited and personal godly power. Even though the religious life of ancient Egypt is depicted as polytheistic, there is an attempt to express, in the different names and forms of the gods, a combination of the names and domains of several different gods in one single god.

The god who is present in his statue and holy animals is a healing and saving god, who, however, punishes people with illness but is also merciful when the ill one turns to him and begs for help and recovery.

Aside from a small number of specific healing gods, there is a large number of gods who have other fountains besides healing, because the request of good health is meant for all gods. Until the end of the New Kingdom, it seems that all ill people, at one time or another, turned to their chosen god, for example to Deir el-Medina, Meret-Seger, or to Amun, who is described in a hymn as the doctor of eye illness. Healing gods accompany people in all their phases, from conception to death.

It was a rich heaven of gods that expected honor, and one constantly had to be on watch so that the "angry crocodile" didn't bite when one least expected it, or so that a delivery was not endangered by demons, or that a weak or sensitive infant was not strained or harmed. Magic could bring illness but could also relieve illness; one had to be immune against the whims of the animal world and the indignation of nature, against being shipwrecked or the results of a difficult desert crossing. Just as important as the correct medicine was the correct "hex"; the best was both.

For this reason, magic-religious sayings in medical treatments pervade the handed-down papyri. They summarize an "integral healing." Papyrus Ebers and Papyrus Hearst, for example, contain a saying the doctor should recite with the instructions of the medications, "I have come out of Heliopolis together with the great one of the large house, the man of protection, the rulers of eternity. And even I have come out of Sais together with the mother of the gods. They have given me their protection... I am one from whom god wants, that he keeps me alive" (Papyrus Ebers 1; 78).

The "Horus-places," with their magical therapy texts, became popular in the course of the dynasty. While one read the texts, the statues, which were to protect against disaster, were doused with water that, when collected, underwent a procedure to become holy water and was used internally as well as externally. This magic therapy was popular, especially in the new dynasty. In Dendera, there were authentic "healing baths" with sinks, where one stretched one's overworked body in the holy medicine water, or at least dunked the ailing body parts in the water, which flowed over the stele.

Once again, we find these calls to the gods in the Papyrus Ebers:

O Isis, great in the art of magic! May you save me, may you free me from all that is bad, evil, and depraved, from disaster by a god or a goddess, from a dead husband or a dead wife, from an enemy who wants to conquer me, just as you redeemed and freed your son Horus. Because I went into the fire and came out of the water, and I do not want to fall into the trap of this day. I have spoken, [and so] I am young....

O Re, speak about your [uräus] snake! Osiris, leave what came out of you! Re speaks about his [uräus] snake! Osiris leaves what came out of him. See, you have saved me from all that is evil, bad, and depraved, from disaster by a god or a goddess, from a dead man or a dead woman...."

And so the text continues.

Naturally, these magical-religious treatments were not only used to drive away evil. They were also much more important when it became necessary to "discuss" poisoning, either the sting of a scorpion or a snake bite. In addition, they were used for eye and skin diseases, burns, "in order to calm the heart, when the legs tremble," for hemorrhoids, aneurisms (to widen the arteries), diseases of the penis, female disorders, to stop menstrual flow, to stimulate breast milk secretion, and for many other "conditions." These conjurations depict a completely legitimate type of therapy; at the same time, medications were administered in order to support the "hex" with drugs. In this way, Papyrus Ebers does not prescribe sayings to "drive a hex out of the stomach," rather the "inside of *hmm*, incense, and *Koloquinten (Citrullus colocynthis)* in sweet beer." Or—to chase away the worst influences of masculine and feminine evilness—a porridge of bread, various fats, honey, bicarbonate, salt, and several other ingredients, which should be made as a compress for diseased parts of the body, are used.

In Papyrus Ebers (no. 733), a cure is described for the *ḥm·t-s wȝ* disease, which is translated word for word as the "art of the protection of magic." The main ingredient of this medicine is an insect's head and its wings prepared in oil. Amazingly enough, there is a modern Egyptian folk medicine cure for hemorrhoids, namely, "a black insect baked in oil, whose head with the entrails have been removed and soaked again in oil at a low temperature" (first noted by C. B. Kluzinger in *Pictures Out of Upper Egypt,* 1877).

The "doctor-magician" implored the most different gods, sometimes only one, but often many. The gods came (or did not come) and drove away the evil spirits that interfered with good health. A request from the Papyrus of London reads: "Suppress yourself, you who comes by arrow [referring to the "arrow of disease"], the gods, who reign in Heliopolis, keep you away."

Occasionally, one also tried to flatter the gods, "Hail to you, Horus, who is the hundredth one in the city, you, the sharp-horned one who shoots at the target . . . I come to you, I prize your beauty. Destroy the illness that sticks in my limbs."

Prayer or conjuration, that is the question here. But that applies for all the magic-religious treatments; even for the magic spells of the Papyrus Berlin:

Early morning spell to read
over a child:
Your arise, O Re,
you arise . . .
I will not give you up,

I will not give the child . . .
My hand lies on,
the seal is your protection.
Re arises.
See, I protect you.

The medical magic spells address single body parts, as if one had the dismemberment of Osiris in mind. And each limb and organ is also often identified with a god:

Your vertex is Re, you healthy child, the back of your head is Osiris, your forehead is Satis, the mistress of Elephantine, your temple is Neith, your eyebrows are the master of the east, your eyes are the master of humanity, your nose is the nourisher of the gods, your ears are the two king's snakes, your elbows are the living sparrow hawk, your arm is Horus, the other is Seth, your . . . is Sopd, the other Nut, the mother of gods . . . your lung is Min . . . your spleen is Suchos, your liver is Harsaphes of Heracleopolis, your entrails are health, your navel is the morning star, your leg is Isis, the other is Nephthys . . . no limb of yours is without a god, every god protects your name and all that comes from you is . . . .

Also, in the *Book of Death* (which we will later discuss in detail) and from *Origines* (AD 300), one finds limb separation and individual gods for each limb. A sensible explanation is that in ancient times, not even the gods were regarded as all-powerful but instead individual gods were associated with one planet or another, this or that river, mountain, straits, or swamp. A mythologically geographical anatomy developed from the personification of the gods; or, stated another way, from the macrocosm "universe" to the microcosm "human." (In this, astrological medicine also plays a role, which we will mention later.)

When we contemplate that the famous scientists like Ranke, Schipperges, or Diepgen were considered to be accurate—and there is no doubt about that—then this report is valid, "Traces of the mythological anatomy remain today in our nomenclature. We call the first cervical vertebra, which carries the head, Atlas, after the Greek demi-god who carried the world. We speak about a mons veneris that lies in the depth of os petrosum. These are not poetic pictures but rather resemblances of an older system that played a large role in the Middle Ages and the Renaissance, and which is not yet dead today ... ." Naturally, in the meantime, we can well imagine how the physician's magic formulas must have affected the treatment of his patients (ie, a placebo effect?). The oral ritual was of eminent meaning and the patient was probably more shocked than the evil spirit. Today we know about the power of suggestion and know how much religious natures appeal to such a treatment. Priests—like physicians—wanted to safely transfer the patient into a frame of mind in which the chances of healing were optimal.

Formulas and medical conjurations whose texts are not in Egyptian also apply. For instance, the Papyrus of London contains four spells in a Semitic dialect and one that must stem from Crete; these are obviously imported formulas that one used for things unfamiliar. Again, parallels are found in the literature of our Middle Ages!

As an example, there is one more conjuration for the plague, with many vague suggestions:

O flame-in-his-face! Rule over the horizon, speak to the head of the Hemsut-house, who allows Osiris, the first of the country, to bloom. O Nachbeth, who lifts the earth to heaven for her father, come, bind the two women around me, around me, to that, which I live and thrive, because I possess the wheat. The first one is the great one, who lives in Heliopolis; the second is Isis; the third is Nephthys; while I am the underling.

O taker of the great one, son of Sakhmet, most powerful of the powerful, son of the disease demon Denad, son of Hathor, the mistress of Krone, and the feeder of streams; when you travel in the heavenly ocean, when you sail in the morning skiff, you have saved me from every disease.

Conjurations for this year, with the breath of every evil wind. Horus, Horus, healthy despite Sakhmet, is for life around all my flesh. Speak the word over two vulture feathers, with which a man has covered himself for protection, wherever he may go. It is protection for the year, which drives out disease in the year of the plague.

A final conjuration formula is added, as it clearly gives an indication for the treating physician; it is to arrest the flow of menstruation, "Anubis has come out, in order to ward off the Nile from entering the shrine, which ... so that its contents are protected. This spell is said over a bound bunch of flax threads. Make a tampon of this, and insert it into her flesh."

Remedies

From the Electric Ray to the Poppy

*More pleasurable is the bread
when the heart is happy,
than richness with sorrow.*
(Lesson from Amenophis, 2400 BC)

The early history of medicine is filled with knowledge and methods of reducing pain. Until 2596 BC, for example, the legendary Huang Tsi, who was known as the "Yellow Emperor," lived in China. He had a personal physician, Nei Ching, who wrote the classical book on acupuncture, which clearly documented how the "energy reservoirs of the body" can be directed in a sensible manner. With bamboo slates and whalebones, he irritated "determined body places" in order to soothe the patient.

Many centuries before this, however, ancient Egyptian physicians tried to cure their patients with many different remedies. Certainly, the most curious remedies are found in the wall drawings of the Fifth Dynasty. From this remote pharaonic time, the *Malapterusus electricus* swam in the Nile and discharged electrical vibrations that were used to provide an "electrical" cure for different types of pain.

Here again, historic literature can replace the omissions in our knowledge: in AD 45, Scribonius Largus described how one cured the pain of gout in ancient Egypt. "When they come, one places a living electric ray *(Torpedo marmorata)* under the foot of the patient. The patient then stands on a wet beach, covered as long as possible with water, until the foot is asleep to the level of the knee."

The same type of "electrotherapy" was recommended for headaches. The scientists Eriksson and Sjölung said in their work *Transcutaneous Nerve Stimulation for Soothing of Pain*:

> Also in the Mediterranean, as in the bordering rivers, one has fish with electrical organs, and one of them was used for therapeutic purposes long before man had methods for the production of electricity.
>
> In the case of the marbled electric ray, the electrical apparatus is present in a modified muscle tissue as embedded plates, which are arranged in columns inside a jelly-type connective tissue. The columns, each with 375 plates, are arranged from the back to the belly and cover the major portion of the anterior part of the body. The many plates in different columns are able to produce enough electrical energy to reach 200 volts. The electric ray grow to be 150 centimeters long and 10 centimeters wide. Probably the specimens used in this "therapy" were not fully grown, so that the discharge would not be so potent.

The electricity produced by these fish changed, of course, with the "build" of their organs. So the *Electrophorus electricus*, the electric eel, a relatively weak fighter, was able to produce a series of rapid discharges (up to sixty per second) but both energy and muscle tired quickly. It needed to pause constantly to re-generate itself and to "recharge its batteries" in order to function perfectly again.

Regarding more unusual medicines, in the tomb of the scribe Userhat of the Eighteenth Dynasty, wall paintings were discovered. There is a physician (or a helper) in a loincloth next to the seated scribe who presses something against his body. At closer view the objects look like cacti, but they are leeches.

The oldest report on leeches known to us comes from the Greek Nikandros, who died in AD 135 in Alexandria and so was of late Hellenic times. Nikandros described how one placed these worms on the body so that the body parts should be freed from blood and congested fluids. The leeches were left in place until they were filled and detached by themselves.

In Egypt this type of treatment had already been known 2,000 years earlier, and artificial "blood letting" was a normal procedure. How it was done—whether, for example, there was an actual opening of the veins with a knife—is not known.

Before we look at the actual recipes in the general pharmacy of Egypt, here are a few abstracts of their curious recipes dealing with gray hair, wrinkles, and body odor. In those days, hairdressers came to the house, unless one had a hairdresser as a permanent employee. Poorer Egyptians were shaved in the shade of the sycamore tree. The "caretaker of the nails and hands and feet and the hair

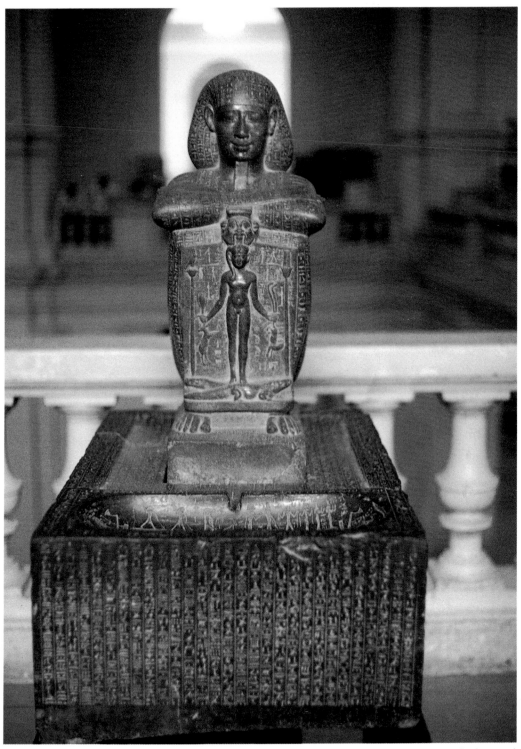

Water was poured over such a "Horus-stele" with serpents and crocodiles while conjuring and health formulas were recited. In this manner the water became healing water. *Egyptian Museum, Cairo.*

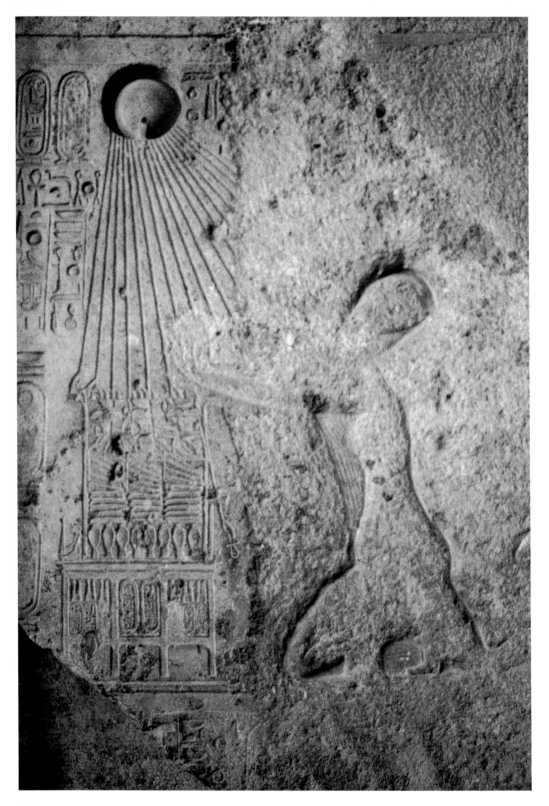

(Left) Akhenaten prays to his god, the sun, and its rays. A relief that can be seen in several places in the Cairo Museum is Akhenaten alone or with his wife and their six daughters. *Egyptian Museum, Cairo.*

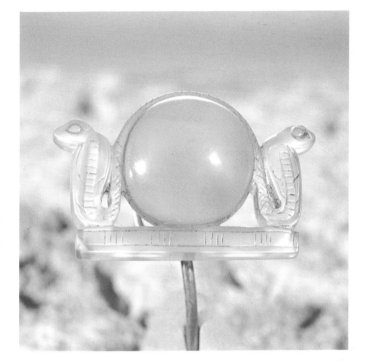

The divine sun god "Re" as amulet with serpents. This particularly lovely piece, which is from the fourth century BC, is made of chalcedony (a cryptocrystalline form of quartz or β-cristabolite and belongs to the group of agates or carneole). This small work of art is only 3.8 centimeters wide. *Schimmel Collection, New York.*

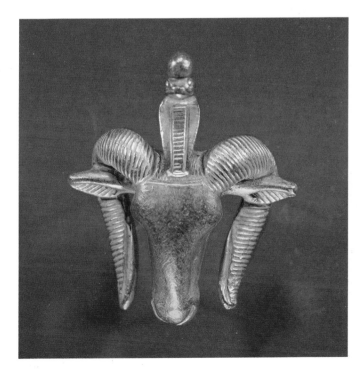

This royal pectoral of gold measures 4.2 centimeters. It was made in the Twenty-fifth Dynasty (about 700 BC). The ram's head as an Amun symbol is represented in many Egyptian temples, famous in the "ram alley" in Karnak. *Schimmel Collection, New York.*

111

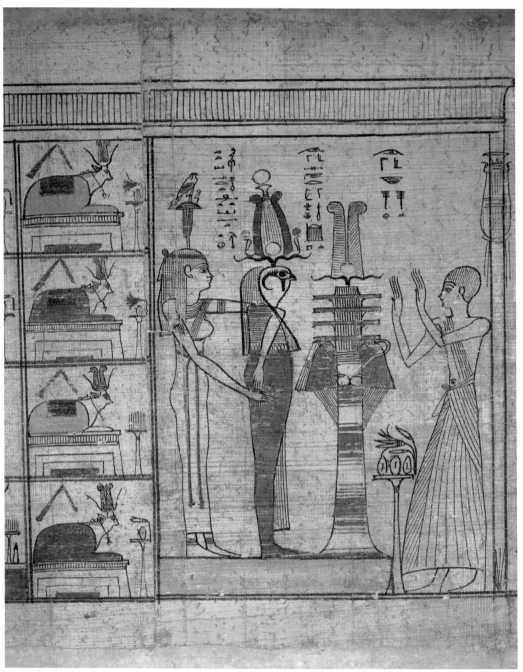

This picture is a cutting from the papyrus *Book of the Dead* in Pajuheru which has a total size of about nine meters. The dead *(right)* prays to Osiris—in the figure of Djed-pillars—the falcon heads, Sokar-Osiris, and Amentet, the goddess of the western dead kingdom. The papyrus originates from the time of the Ptolemaic Dynasty. In ancient Egypt at about 1500 BC, a *Book of the Dead* belonged in each tomb, either painted on the wall or as papyrus. The prettiest papyri were found in the tombs of Ani, Hunefer, and Anahi in Thebes. *State Collection of Egyptian Art, Munich.*

attendant" would bring his own hair-growing recipe from his personal store. The medicine to counteract baldness was made from the oil of the boxthorn. The plant is called "helba" in Arabic and is used in many remedies today.

Once more, the Papyrus Ebers offers information about the conditions of Egyptian cosmetics, "One part each of rubber or turpentine [pistachio tree], wax, fresh ben oil [from the nut of the *Moringa*, a plant similar to the poppy], and Cyprus grass are finely ground, placed in the juice of the plants, and applied daily to the face. This removes wrinkles in the face." For dry skin, the papyrus indicates: "Bile from cattle, oil, rubber, and ostrich egg-flour are mixed, diluted with plant juice, and used daily for washing the face."

One must go far back in time if one wants to know of the medicines and their application. At the University of Göttingen, for a long time it was sought and then discovered that the selection of medications was based on the principle of "similia similibus curantur" ("likes are cured by likes"). And only long-term experimental testing would provide the experience to differentiate between effective drugs and those that had no effect or were injurious. There were certain medications so bold as "to glue the fracture of the outside of the skull with the pulverized shell of an ostrich" or to treat migraines with the "cooked skull of a siluroid." Some recipes have the concluding statement,

"million times proved," or indicate a long-gone royal period. These are often remedies that were first used as magic but were later crystallized in "experience medicine" as being effective.

On the other hand, there are exact lists of possible "single drugs" that can originate from any source: from the mineral kingdom, or the world of plants, and—naturally—based on parts or secretions of animals or humans. A common list consists of eggs, excrement, fat, hair, honey, leather, liver, meat, milk, skin, testicles, tongue, tooth, urine, and wax. The animals include the bat, cat, crocodile, donkey, fish, fly, frog, goat, goose, hippopotamus, lion, lizard, locust, mouse, ostrich, pelican, ram, turtle, snake, swallow, scorpion, and siluroid. Also, the plant kingdom includes blossoms, leaves, roots, stalks, fruits and resins, oil, rubber, myrrh, poppy (we will discuss opium later), dates, dill, peas, barley, pomegranate, sycamore, tamarisk, and onions. Finally, the mineral kingdom includes water, agate, alum, carnelian, copper, flint, iron, lapis lazuli, lead, malachite, ocher, pumice, salt, and sodium carbonate. And besides these, products such as breads, beer, and wine were commonly used.

The Egyptian professor of history Dr Ali Hassan said at a conference in Cairo, "Twelve different types of headache were treated with a variety of drugs [and combinations of drugs] according to the papyri. Also used were coriander, laudanum, tamarisk, sodium bicarbonate, stone pine, incinerated fish bones, goose feet, and also fruits that we are no longer able to identify. We also discovered a number of medications for diseases of the ears. At least five of them are rational and so have nothing to do with magic. They are made up of plants and minerals, in an oil base with malachite."

Crocodiles and antibiotics

"When age comes, the soul flies like birds to the days of childhood." This sentence was written by Sinuhe in his recollections. He was well able to remember the days of his childhood: those were the days of the toy wooden crocodiles that he rattled through the streets and which his father, the physician, had received as payment for treatment from the carpenter of the pharaoh. A toy crocodile was only available to royal children.

Let us sit for a short while with the small Sinuhe in the sand and wait for the water. From the four-room house, constructed out of Nile mud and bricks, there was a small terrace and a pond, "the stony basin," shadowed by a sycamore. The garden was only a few paces wide, and toward the street there were acacia bushes under which Sinuhe liked to rest and spy on the wide world. In those days, it was the height of luxury if one had a small pond in the garden, maybe

with palms or fig trees and with grape vines and flowers used for table decorations. In a land with such a hot climate, the people lived on the street. The poorest of the poor slept on a bundle in a dusty alley. Those who were moderately poor had grass huts, which are similar to those inhabited today by the shepherds of Egypt. The next step up was the brick hut made of Nile mud. This porous material is still considered by the "average people" of today as the best construction material. The rich preferred multilevel "atrium houses" such as the Roman and the Spanish in which the rooms overlook the atrium. These houses had up to seventy rooms and could have as many as five floors.

There, the small Sinuhe, who was to become a physician like his father, played with his tame Ichneumon (a viverrid) and a little monkey. There was an incredible perfume: from the Nile came waves of cedar- and myrrh-scented air and the beer breath of the sea travelers. There was the smell of fish being fried in oil and —when pretty women passed by—of ointments and roses, and in general, all the good smells of the Orient. When his father finally arrived with his medical bag there was the smell of strong ointments and bitter medications on his garments and sometimes even worse smells. This was because the physician also cured with lizard filth, gazelle dung, and the things that a crocodile digests. Fish bile and crushed cow liver were (and still are) used against infection and inflammations. "Dirty apothecary" is the name given by the medical historians of today to this medication treasury, which is still being used in the twentieth century. Urine was used for washing; mud and earth were used in bandages.

Regarding mud—the key word of "Egyptian Medicine and its Curing"—in 1948, Dr Benjamin M. Duggar, who for twenty-one years had been professor of plant physiology at the University of Wisconsin, surprised the world with the medicine Aureomycin, which today is used successfully to cure trachoma. Aureomycin was the newest among the so-called antibiotic miracle drugs (of which penicillin was the first). The story of its discovery sounds funny, as if it were from the tales of the 1001 nights; however, scientifically it is reality. Duggar and his co-workers studied the soil of a cemetery located close to the university, and between 1944 and 1946, approximately 30,000 soil types were studied. Only in the soil of the cemetery did they find a growth of fungus that destroyed disease-producing bacteria in the same manner as other mold fungi, for example, penicillin.

Here the circle is complete: research proves that filth and urine excreted by humans can contain effective antibiotics. The "dirt apothecary" of the old Egyptians, of the Middle Ages, and of the nineteenth century was completely correct in his evaluation of the effectiveness of soil, and subsequent cures were not due to

chance or miracle. Only the Papyrus Ebers gives us information of at least fifty-five recipes having to do with human excretion.

The Papyrus Ebers also describes important medications that only came to light after better understanding of vitamins. Honey and beer were considered a means of administering medicine. In this, the physicians were ahead of their time—especially because they recommended the "sediment" as a drug against intestinal complaints and skin diseases. Today we know that yeast is rich in vitamin B and also contains antibiotics useful against abscesses, sores, and boils.

There is always the mention of bread in the medications of pharaonic times. This must be explained because what is meant is "rotting bread," or bread that is moldy. It was considered the best remedy against blisters, intestinal diseases, and suppurating wounds. "The physician should fight against diseases and not get out of their way" are the words from a text from the Middle Kingdom. The discovery and development of antibiotics allows us to clarify how much "experience" the Egyptians already had. They knew of the anti-infectious properties of molds 4,000 years ago!

Earlier (in the chapter "Introduction") mention was made of a "radish strike" during the pyramid construction. Even here there is an underlying medical reason. We resort to Herodotus again, who noticed: "On the pyramid it is noted the number of radishes, garlic, and onions the workers should receive. If what the translator told me is correct, about 1,600 silver talents were spent." By today's reckoning, this would be about ten million dollars.

For a long time researchers did not understand this enormous expense for the distribution of garlic and onions; even physicians could give no insight. This changed in 1948, when Karrer and Schmidt produced Raphanin. This is a product obtained from the seeds of radishes that has antibiotic properties against bacteria such as cocci and coli. Similarly discovered in radish juice, then in garlic and in onions, were Allicin and Allistatin, which are effective against dysentery, typhus, and cholera.

With this in mind, it becomes understandable why the pharaohs did not deny daily radish rations to their workers, and why workers and priests protested. Ramses III had to help his peasants quickly when communication came from the construction workers of the necropolis of Thebes and, according to the Papyrus Turin, they complained, "We came because we are hungry and thirsty. We have no dresses, we have no ointments...we have no vegetables."

Each worker received, for example, in Wadi Hammamat at the time of King Senwosret I, a daily ration of ten breads, one-third jar of beer, and a water sack. The specialized worker was happy with his twenty breads and one-half jar of beer. In later times, under Ramses IV, workers had ten breads, three jars of beer, two units of meat, and three cakes.

The ancient Egyptians took great pleasure in eating and drinking; we will return to this later.

The early physicians were especially careful with the dosages of their medicines. Medications taken orally were not only prescribed in cakes, porridge, gruel, or in pill form but as beverages, ointments for rubbing, or as cones for the anus and vulva. They were carefully measured, particularly with expensive drugs such as incense and poppy (meconium or laudanum), which were used to relieve pain or during operations. Only the Greeks called the milky product of the poppy "opion" from "opos" (plant juice). Opium (currently termed) contains several alkaloids: morphine, noscapine, codeine, papaverine, and thebaine. The Egyptians probably obtained it from Asia Minor. They also had to travel far for incense, which was considered a medication and used for embalming. The mixture of myrrh, olibanum, benzoe, storax, and tolu-balsam made the Saba and the Minae in South Arabia wealthy people.

The number of drugs of which ancient Egyptian physicians had knowledge of constitutes more than a third of the medications used today. Whether it is the Christmas rose or turpentine of the spruce— industry uses the experience of the Egyptians. We know of a medical text in which there is talk of *spnn* and *spn*.

Even with careful translation, we are talking about a drug that is both good and bad and is unknown in modern medicine: once again, it is the poppy.

For a long time researchers doubted that the Egyptians really knew of the opium poppy and the effective components in the milky juice of the unripe fruit. If they had only read their Homer carefully! The extraordinary wealth of drugs in Egypt is described in the Odyssey. The crying Telemachus who receives from Helen a "forgetting drink," which was certainly poppy juice, is described. Homer reports on this with the words: "Such witchcraft medicines had she, the daughter of the gods, potent, which were given to her by the wife of Thot, Polydamna, an Egyptian." It is the first report on the theme of opium in the history of medicine.

From the darkness of history we find another medicine in the bright light of today's research: *Mandragora* (mandrake), a plant that for centuries was part of many different myths. With the Egyptians and late into the Middle Ages, "Alraune" was used as a narcotic in operations. In our day, it was discovered that the double-rooted plant (Nefertiti in a drawing is shown placing it next to her husband's mouth) contains atropine and scopolamine, drugs used to place a patient in a twilight sleep during an operation. Scopolamine and atropine come from the nightshade family, and both are found in plants such as belladonna (*Atropa bella-*

donna), henbane (folia hyoscyami mutici) or the *Datura*, the thorn apple. These small plants with beautiful flowers were known as "drugs of the physicians."

Early Indians were also familiar with these drugs, as were the monks of the Middle Ages and the ancient Egyptians. The thorn apple contains arthrop alkaloid, flavonoid glycoside, nicotine, and cumarin. Misuse is deadly. Four to five grams of the raw leaves are enough to cause death. In 1869, the clergy in Paris noted the mishap of a "respected member" who had been bit by a rabid dog. At the worst point of thirty hours of cramps, he was given a "pinch of *Datura*." He was to eat the leaves and swallow them, after which the poor priest fell into "spasmodic convulsions" and delirium; the next day he awoke healthy.

Similar reports can be read in Egyptian medicine, although thorn apple medication was only used after Christ's birth. In the year 36 BC, the Roman Antonius went to battle against the people of Parther in Asia Minor. They wrote proudly about the effects of their plants, "The troops had to take their refuge in roots and herbs that they were not familiar with. So they encountered an herb that kills after making one mentally ill. Those who ate of it forgot what they had done so far and did not recognize anything." It was *Datura* or the thorn apple. It is thought that the priests of Apollo's temple in Delphi ate those leaves to prepare themselves for the ceremonies of forecasting. It is certain that the Incas brewed a *Datura* drink to get closer to their gods. They prepared it in the sun temple at Sagomozo from the seeds (it was called "Floripondio").

Still another remedy, the tropical Galant, together with pepper, was brought to Egypt from explorations. It was used as a medication for various heart conditions. Through laboratory research, it was discovered that cypress grass (galanga) and pepper contain agents that are active for heart problems. A thin oil can avoid lump formation of each little leaf. In case of heart infarct due to a damaged blood vessel wall, this drug can alter the thrombus that is closing the blood vessel.

It is not possible to estimate how many Egyptians had access to these drugs and how many paid for their effects with their lives. Early on, slaves were probably experimented on, and also prisoners received drugs until they were rendered unconscious. Certainly, however, from what we read in the literature, the Egyptians had a very good idea about the mortality potential and the curative effects of the drugs when they were dosed properly. For the first time in the history of medicine, at the Nile, exact measurements were taken and Egyptian physicians also knew the dosage of nonpoisonous drugs. From kingdom to kingdom and from dynasty to dynasty, the recipes became perfected. This also explains why, in medical papyri, the weight of a drug is no longer given; it is assumed to be part of the experience and knowledge of a progressive medical profession.

Measurement units were calculated according to different systems. However, they apparently were all based on the bushel. A bushel was 4.785 liters, and the smallest part of this was the "ro"—the 320th part of the bushel or about fifteen cubic centimeters (a full tablespoon). So, for example, the recipe for the "elimination of the fever" says: "Powder from dates, 5 ro, powder from *d3rt*, 5 ro, liquid porridge, 40 ro, will be cooked until about 30 ro fluid remains. You shall give it to a man or a woman when the heart is endurable until he gets well ...." Although Egyptian physicians knew the dosages and manner of administration, for us the "miraculous porridge" remains a riddle, for instance, the fact that it was necessary to leave medication for the abdomen in the dew overnight and then to take it for four days. External medication was simpler. For rubbing, one prepared creams with olive oil, ricinus, and animal fat. In the Papyrus Ebers, a local use of an astringent (this medical expression is used for the inflammation-hindering effects of "gathering-together" substances) against rectal prolapse is described as follows: "For a displacement of the back part: myrrh, incense, reed nut from the garden, *mhtt* from the river bank, celery, coriander, oil, and salt are cooked together, placed on cotton and put in the rear end."

Suppositories used by Egyptian physicians for the intestines or vagina had binders of oil, milk, or beer. And with enemas, usually a half to one liter and a half was introduced. They were associated with mild drugs which probably were supposed to be held or absorbed in a natural way to produce elimination. According to Pliny (Roman scholar, AD 23–19), the white-headed ibis, the sacred bird, by using his long, curved bill, was able "to clean each part, by which he is very healthy, to eliminate the backlog of his nutrition."

Many medications had to be taken for four consecutive days and at the right time of the year such as sawdust of stone pine or grapes. The Papyrus Hearst contains recipes against the bad smell of sweat in summer, and the Berlin Papyrus describes the remedy against a disease (of which we know nothing) "that happens in winter to all articulations." Such remedies are often used in combination. Hence, one rubbed against the "rose in the abdomen(?)" a cream of turpentine, wax, and four other (unknown) components, and ordered with it a laxative of colocynth and senna. The combination was drunk. The enema was particularly the order of the day in the Papyrus Chester Beatty.

The ox was "man's best friend" in ancient Egypt since it not only worked but also provided nourishment, skin, fire materials, and drugs. Its brain, liver, spleen, bile, blood, marrow, meat, and fat were used for medicinal purposes. Compared to it, the brain of the siluroid fish created medications of small value. Swallow's liver was used by Egyptian women to overcome weakness; "dried, pounded and with tough liquid of fermented beverage," it was placed on the chest and the abdomen of a woman who had experienced a miscarriage.

In summary, the old texts mention the use of a number of curative drugs and lethal poisons, from magnesium to antimony—the poisonous stibnite. The latter was found in a cosmetic box dating about 2500 BC. To be exact, the name for it is red stibnite because of its cherry red crystals, but gray stibnite was more commonly used.

A short digression into medicinal history may be useful. The Old Kingdom was already 4,000 years past when fight and discord occurred on the European medical clinic scene. The reason was that antimony, under the name emetic tartar, was making people crazy. It was prescribed against leprosy, malaria, chest disease, and many other diseases. French physicians tore their hair in worry until it was certain that the young king, Louis XIV, had cured himself from typhus with antimony preparations (the name at the time was stibium). There was, and there is no antimony in Egypt. We know this from the writings about Hatshepsut. However, today it is even in the matches.

The uterus of the cat, antimony sulfide, yellow ocher, sodium carbonate, alabaster powder, or ink extract with charcoal and resin, rubber and red sand used against mouth inflammations and in diarrhea were "pharmaceuticals" that the Egyptian physician was able to prepare at home. There were no pharmacists. One collected, saved, and searched—possibly instinctively—for the medicines. The knowledge that can be attributed to the physicians of the pharaohs is of extremely high quality. If one disregards subcutaneous, intramuscular, and intravenous injections and operative possibilities, it is amazing what Imhotep, Hesi Re, and all others were able to accomplish as they came out from under the shadow of the tamarisk.

Organ therapy has been known to physicians for a long time. For 4,000 years, treatment of sterility with sex gland tissue (indifferent as to which sex) has been known. Particularly because there was high child mortality in ancient Egypt, impotence and sterility were considered a great shame. Only the potent, rich person could afford to have his loved one delay pregnancy for one or two years and have her use contraception (see the chapter "Love, Lust, and Birth").

The literature does not definitely say how, 3,000 or 4,000 years ago at the Nile, one used the testicles of the common otter and beaver. However, one can assume it was done as in the Middle Ages with the expensive castoreum. Almost every dictionary explains to us what that meant. For example, in the Brockhous travel guide: "Beaver musk, exchange products from the beaver, resin gloss, brown bulk in two long brown sacs covered with skin (beaver sacs) next to the sex glands. Castoreum smells very intensely as sweet animal leather and is used today in the perfume industry...."

Put simply, beaver musk is a material that is separated from animals of either sex into sacs between the sex parts and the anus. From the male through the blood-vessel-rich foreskin, and from the female above the clitoris are obtained bitter principle, resins, fats, and acids (this can be explained by the nutrition of the beaver, namely tree bark).

Castoreum became famous among the Islamic physicians and the descendants of the Egyptians (ie, the physicians of the Coptics) for its calming and cramp-soothing action. Misuse, "which the midwives not infrequently resort to in order to expedite labor," is urgently warned about.

Creative sleep as remedy

As has been demonstrated with old Egyptian tales as well as biblical stories, the gods appear to mortals primarily during sleep and in dreams. However, during the Middle Kingdom, dreaming was studied as a science, and the curative remedy of sleep was "discovered." It was primarily curative for priests and in the temples.

Three thousand years before the theories of Sigmund Freud on neurosis were recognized, the Egyptians believed in a spontaneous dream as opposed to a provoked, looked-for dream. This required that one give oneself to the gods in the temples of the times and be led to the "rapture of sleep." The priest-physicians were sure they could cure certain diseases in this manner.

The favorite places for curative sleep for which pilgrims came from far way were Deir el-Medina, the "sanatorium" in Dendera Abydos, the side rooms of the Sethos temple, and the Serapeum in Memphis. Adrian de Buck and Serge Sauneruon were interested in this early curative psychology and wrote extensively on the subject.

Body Maintenance and Care

Hygiene and Circumcision

*Scared of God, they all are, in all measures
and they have strange customs.
They drink from cups that they
wash, they use dresses
which are cleaned daily,
they prefer to be clean than
wealthy. And they do not kiss each other
after having eaten."*

(Herodotus)

The history of medicine of the pharaohs forces us to think about how matters of religion affected attention to the body and hygiene; there was great concern for maintenance and care of the body before the last trip to mummification and the journey to the other world.

Before stepping onto the "sun boat," which took the person to Osiris, the body had to be in good condition. This required certain rules of a hygienic nature, which even found their way into biblical history. Moses also took with him knowledge of the local medicines when he, in 1330 BC, led a large number of people from Egypt into the Promised Land. Before the legendary man from the tribe of Levi went on the way to Mount Sinai (Horeb) and received the Ten Commandments, a forty-year trip, he preached—as a student of

Egyptian physicians—principles of hygiene, among them, circumcision.

Much has been written since that time about the most common surgical intervention in medical history for boys or youths, and much of it is nonsense. In Egypt, boys between the sixth and the twelfth year (and this is still the custom in other countries) were circumcised. Was this practiced for religious or hygienic reasons? Even the experts ask.

One of the old masters of Egyptian research, Henry Sigerist, quotes Herodotus: "He writes that the Egyptian introduced circumcision for hygienic reasons, because they put cleanliness above prudishness, a conclusion that certainly is wrong! The operation took place in the temple with a stone knife, which tells us how old the custom is."

"Possibly," it continues, "it is ritual initiation" (the age of manhood is considered here), and it continues, "we know from old manuscripts that blood fell from the phallus of the god" (ie, Re) "as he mutilated himself. The circumcision is a copy of the unsuccessful operation of the god. However it may be, there is little doubt of the religious aspects."

The author of this book also does not believe this any more than did the famous historian Adolf Erman, who judged circumcision in the following manner: "It was introduced totally for hygienic principles." And in this he was correct, as medicine today demonstrates. We are aware of a serious disease known as balanitis. In hot climates, in which desert sand can clog our ears, other parts of the body are also affected. Balanitis is a purulent inflammation of the glands in men and of the internal prepuce. The sandy desert wind attacks uncircumcised men, in particular those who are only wearing a caftan, a gallabejja, or a djellaba, causing a health hazard. In early Egypt, this fact was considered a cause of male infertility. Since then, circumcision has been performed and balanitis has been avoided.

According to Jewish tradition, circumcision is considered a special covenant made between Abraham and God. Today among Arabs, it is considered a form of "coming of age." Scientists consider circumcision a substitution for communion or confirmation, but this latter reasoning is also nonsense. The descendants of the ancient Egyptians—Copts—were circumcised and baptized in the Christian faith. Circumcision was for hygiene, baptism was for the soul and spirit.

Following is another theory, which often appears in psychological litanies: circumcision, it is said, is the opposite of castration and is a means of condemning and preventing incest. Comment about this is probably unnecessary.

In the medical papyri there is no mention of circumcision. There are, however, representations of the two available techniques. One technique can be seen in two different phases in the tomb of Ankh-ma-Hor

(Old Kingdom, Sixth Dynasty). The physician rubs the penis of the young men with a cream; the written text says that this is "so that it can be tolerated [does not hurt]." To his assistant, he says, "Hold him well, so that he does not fall down." To which the answer is, "I do what you tell me so that you will praise me." The physician then cuts lengthwise.

The other depiction of circumcision is from the time of the New Kingdom. The surgeon pushes the foreskin downward with his finger and holds his knife crosswise over the surgical area. Today it is certain that before Egyptian men undertook the trip into the sacred land, they not only considered circumcision a sensible procedure, but also a cleansing regulation.

Egyptians also considered food laws to be measures of ensuring health for the long journey. Forbidding pork meat, for example, which is referred to by the Greeks in the same breath as circumcision, is information enough to connect hygienic reasons to both. Experience had shown clearly to biblical families and their Egyptian ancestors that fat, rich meat breeds rottenness and spoilage in hot climates—it is called dyspepsia today and causes vomiting spells. The effects in southern heat are far worse than those in northern and middle European climates. More than in other regions, there are also parasitic diseases such as those caused by taeniae (tapeworms) and trichinosis. The latter appears in initial stages as harm-less, but with muscle or intestinal involvement it can lead to respiratory paralysis.

The Egyptians considered the pig to be a dirty animal. Whoever touched it would be sick unless he bathed immediately in the Nile.

"The pig herder cannot come into the temple," noticed Herodotus on an Egyptian trip, "also, no one can give to them their daughter. They are the abomination of the gods" (with the exception of two gods who received pig sacrifices).

Pigs were sacrificed to Dyonysius and the moon goddess, always at full moon. When the pig was killed, the tip of the tail, the retina, the spleen, and bacon were placed in a heap and burned. The rest had to be eaten during the night.

Here the circle on religion is closing as are their food laws. The Old Testament says, (Lev. 11:7) "and the swine...he is unclean to you...." And also (Deut. 14:3, 8), "thou shalt not eat any abominable thing.... And the swine...is unclean unto you: ye shall not eat of their flesh, nor touch their dead carcase." In the Koran, the food laws which take care of health restrictions sound very similar ("As is explained to the believers and the Christians," Book VI, 146).

The beginning of the oldest original religious cultures and their health rules are, as has already been said, based on the ancient Egyptian and pharaonic times.

The belief of the divine origin of each body part forced the ancient Egyptians to a strong control and care of body. Every body part had a "protective god." That is clearly understood in the Egyptian *Book of the Dead* (see the chapter "The Trip to the Other Side") in saying 42, which says:

My hair is [the god] Nun,
My spirit is Re [the sun],
My eyes are Hathor,
My ears are Upuaut.
My nose is the territory of Letopolis,
My lips are Anubis,
My teeth are Selkis,
My neck is the goddess, Isis.
My arms are Ba from Mendes,
My breast is Neith, the mistress of Sais.
My back is Seth,
My penis is Osiris.
My meat is the mistress of Cheraha,
My body and my spinal column are
   Sakhmet,
My backside is Horus-eye . . .
My foot is Ptah.
No part is without a god.
Thoth is the protector of my whole body,
Of Re I am all the time.

Priests in ancient Egypt shaved their entire body every third day in order to avoid lice. They bathed twice a day and two times each night, had to constantly wash their linen clothes, and were only allowed to wear "shoes from Byblos," which were reed sandals. "Thousands of uses they had to observe" wrote Herodotus. For this they had at their disposal cellars filled with geese, cattle meat, dried fish, and wine, which they could use to fill the body according to their own disposition.

How they occupied themselves with their digestion is a favorite theme of historical literature. (Even Herodotus could not help himself in writing that "the Egyptians empty their intestines inside the houses, the urine is emanated by the men in a sitting position, the women standing.") In any case, the ancient Egyptians had at their disposal perfectly connected toilet facilities—even in simple households. Mummified pharaohs were sent in "perched position" into the tomb for voyage into the next life.

In 31 BC, the Roman military technician Vitrubius Pollio composed ten architecture books (important works for the builders of the Renaissance) in which it is written that around 2500 BC there were, in Abusir, bath facilities that were 400 meters long, with astounding copper tubing.

About 1,000 years later in El Amarna, the bust of Nefertiti was discovered (and can be seen in Berlin today), at the same time wonderful bath facilities were found that were also used with "curative waters" for medicinal purposes.

About 1370 BC, the city Akhetaten (El Amarna) was founded by the Pharaoh Amenophis IV (already discussed as the "heretic king," Akhenaten). In this rapidly decaying capital (this was discovered, in the meantime, by excavation) there were public toilet facilities with shady street entrances. They were flooded at night and the waters were drained into canals. Construction plans for small houses (worker colonies) in the "planned city" of the revolutionary king documents the existence of washrooms and abortive ones or small bathing rooms. Amenophis IV had clear ideas about hygiene. He was sure that infective diseases and contagious diseases had to be fought or they would disseminate many times over, especially in small places.

The usual one-family house of Imhotep or Sobure was, of course, small in size. But even so, each family had sanitary facilities at the time when Europeans did their eliminating behind a tree, and where in Rome, people took a bath in rain showers. The Egyptians used long copper-tubing systems that ended, obviously, in the Nile. Unfortunately, this created a dilemma. The Nile did not only bring fruitful mud, it also was used as "drainage." After the flooding returned to its course, if the water puddles remained, they became breeding grounds for flies. And, if the canals were not cleaned properly, malaria developed.

Particularly under Turkish domination, sanitation became very bad. Napoleon found this too during his Egyptian stay, "In no other land has the administration such an influence on the well-being of everyone. The administration is good, so the canals are carefully kept in good condition, and orders are followed carefully."

In any case, conditions were ideal for the development of every type of insect. Herodotus also commented about this in his description of his trips, "Against the mosquitoes, which are in immense quantities, use the following measures: those who live above the marshes are saved, since they go up and sleep and since the mosquitoes are unable to fly high because of the winds. However, those who live in the marshes should use the following in spite of the columns: each should have a net to fish during the day, at night he needs it for resting. He puts the net up and crawls underneath and sleeps under it. If he covers himself with a dress or a cloth the mosquitoes go underneath and bite. With the net they do not try."

When the Nile with its high waters brought its mud, it brought germs responsible for the many "Egyptian diseases." The worst was schistosomiasis, which is bilharziasis, and in today's Egypt is called "Billy the hook worm." Today, people at the Nile can laugh about this, but it was not so funny 5,000 years ago any more than it is today. Forty percent of all Egyptians are infested with this type of larvae, which develops in the body over many years. This microscopic worm penetrates the body through the walls of the intestine and causes growth of the tissues of the large intestine while other, sexually mature worms enter the liver. There they wait for a chance to "attack," which they do when the body is weakened by an infection of some sort. Or, they take long enough to develop tumors of the liver, which will kill the victim. The host animals of these worms are snails that swim in the

Nile. A few years ago, the wife of the murdered former president of Egypt, Jehan Sadat, tried to champion large poison treatment in order to fight these snails, but it was not a success.

Today, if one sees a peasant on the banks of the Nile washing himself, one can be certain that he is already carrying the disease, of which texts say that it "does devastation to small children." Naturally, children play daily on the banks of the Nile.

So keep your foot on board during your trip on the river, do not dangle it overboard. There are no more crocodiles and hippopotami, but the hookworm comes silently and deadly.

Even though they knew of this danger, the beautiful people of the Nile—often for religious reasons—bathed in the stream. The men did not welcome this type of hygiene, but for the women two statements were important, "You should bathe before each meal and also wash your teeth." For this type of washing, one had different types of containers and different types of cans, for example, for feet and hands. In the ruins of a house of the Late Period, a container was found with the inscription: "You can wash your face in well-being and health. Be happy, heart!"

The hymn to the sun from Amarna, which was written many centuries ago says: "In the morning the people awake and get on their feet, because you [sun] did not let them get up. Their body will be washed and they take their clothes,

their arms are lifted in their prayers, because you appeared." In the necropolis of Thebes, a text can be found that says: "The dead washes himself when Re appears," that is, when the sun appears.

Those who had no servants lathered themselves with a soap-type paste, or with sodium carbonate or soda. Psychologists have discovered that the less clothes people wear, the more likely they are to take care of their bodies. If this is pertinent to any group of people, it is to the Egyptians. All types of creams and aromatic oils were considered in all levels of the population as almost unaffordable luxury items, which still one rubbed with delight on one's body. One wanted to "smell oneself" in the truest meaning of the word.

The men in the Ancient Kingdom wore small beards and shaved themselves once a day. Body hair was not considered desirable. The ladies of ancient Egypt shaved themselves with bronze knives with great care and used thin tweezers to eliminate undesired hair. We have already discussed how they treated their eyes. However, the care that was taken with body hair still needs description. The hair of the Egyptians was black, and it was taboo to show it graying. Loss of hair and baldness brought shame. Against it, one oiled one's head with the blood of a black calf, oxen, or the fat of a black snake, fat from hippopotamus or crocodile, or the burned spikes of a hedgehog. In this regard, the ancient Egyptians were not ahead

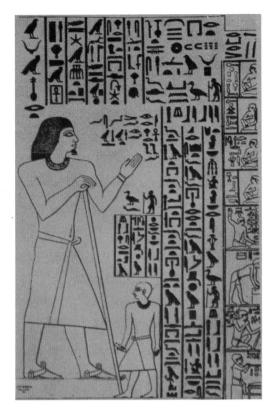

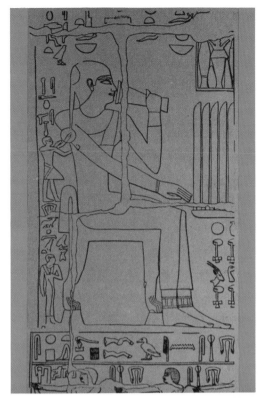

(Above left) The wall designs were found in Giza in the mastaba of Nefertiti (Fifth Dynasty). Fifteen persons, among them widows, are represented, and the uppermost person is Nefer-Hor-en Ptah, who is simply described as "physician." The large figure should represent the king himself, the small ones his son Ipty.

(Above right) Seshem-Nefer (his tomb found in Saqqara) was "inspector of the physicians" and was well informed about all drugs, for example, the thorn apple *(Datura) (right)*. Two leaves of this tropical plant can kill a child. In ancient Egypt (later also in South America) it was cultivated as a drug and worked up as a medication.

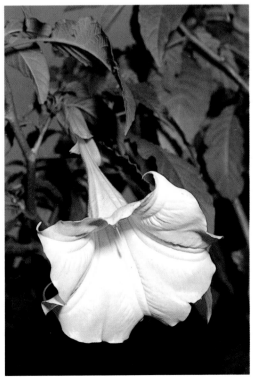

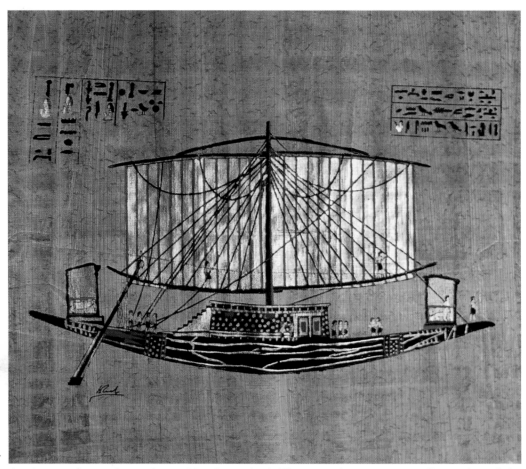

A papyrus of a sun barge (owned by the author). These sun barges supposedly conducted the dead person on the trip to the other world. The tombs show many types of these boats. They were drawn according to prehistoric rafts and were steered with two oars. They were decorated with two sacred eyes (udjat eyes) on the bow and color ledges on the hull. On the deck planks, painted white, there was a gold throne for the god. These boats were used by pharaohs in "real" life. About twenty years ago, next to the pyramid of Khufu (Cheops) the sun barge of the pharaoh was found and is now in a wooden hall in Giza, 4,500 years later. Also, on the inside wall of the second golden vault of Tutankhamun, texts and pictures of the sun barge were found. The Egyptians associated the travel of the sun in the sky with the travel of the god Re, who ruled over the sky waters. This concept is only understandable in a land in which the river is the only means of transportation. In the dead text appears the wish to be with Re, and to accompany him. This is both a participation of world rule and the highest achievement in the other world for the pharaoh.

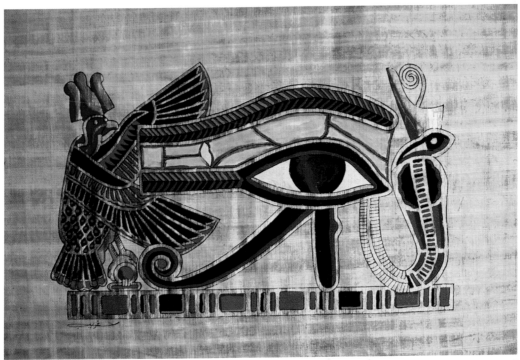

(Above) Udjat eye (eye of the light god, Horus), symbol of cyclic renewal of life and made of three parts: the human eye, the eyelids of the falcon, and the eyebrow of the predatory cat.
(Below) Circumcision papyrus. *New papyri, owned by author.*

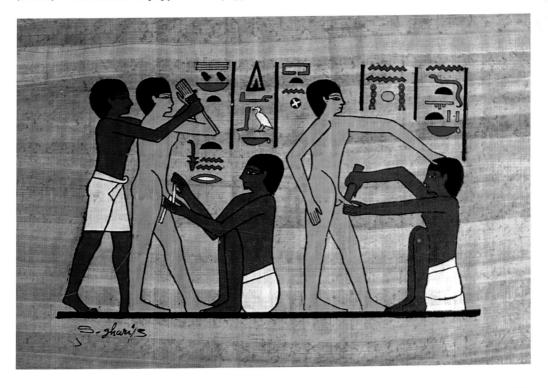

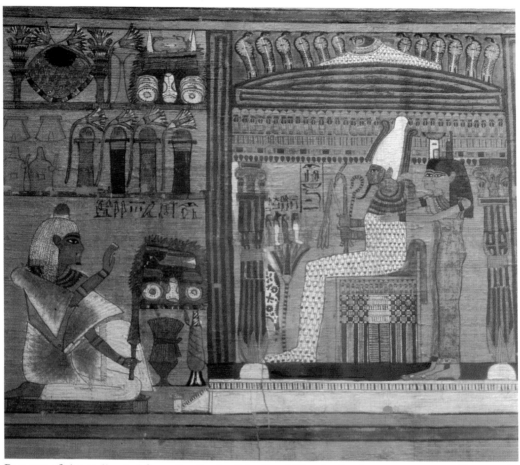

Papyrus of the scribe Ani from the *Book of the Dead*. The dead, who presents a sacrifice, sits in front of Osiris, the ruler of the kingdom of the dead, who is sitting on a throne (the papyrus is dated from the Nineteenth Dynasty). Osiris himself was murdered in the Nile after a bitter intrigue and later was cut in pieces. His sister and wife, Isis, searched all over Egypt for his corpse parts, which were then—according to legend—placed together. From then on, Osiris was the main god of the underworld. *British Museum, London.*

of us; their methods were not any more successful than ours.

What holds the body and soul together

Our knowledge of the foods of ancient Egypt is derived primarily from representations in tombs. There we find hunting scenes in the delta or pictures of Egyptians making bread, brewing beer, killing animals, and the presentation of sacrifices. Egyptians ate balanced, healthy meals.

The main foods of the simple people were bread and fish. About fifty different varieties of breads were known. The variations were not only due to the use of different types of flour and their mixture but also due to the refining of the flour, and unsweetened or honey-containing dough. In the delta, there was even a type of bread made with dried lotus. The flour often contained many impurities of chaff and sand. Therefore, abrasion during mastication was a cause for the bad teeth of the Egyptians. Besides flat cakes there was a cone-shaped bread. The baker heated a conical form, and when it was hot he covered it with dough without putting it in the fire again. It rose but would not burn.

Vegetables and fruits were available in quantity, particularly garlic, onions, different types of beans, gourds, cucumbers, olives, figs, dates, leeks, and melons. For cooking fat, olive oil is used.

Meat dishes were not eaten daily. They were considered special occasion food in spite of the fact that cattle had been bred since the beginning of Egyptian history, and bred to excess in the New Kingdom. In this manner, one had food: milk and—particularly draft—animals. Also, there were goats and sheep. These were primarily for food because there was no need for wool.

Fowl of any kind was greatly appreciated. Chasing a duck with a boomerang was a favorite activity among wealthier people. Wine was only present on the tables of the rich. Besides water and milk, beer was the favorite drink of the Egyptians. It was always talked about in a lively, often exaggerated manner. Drunkenness was apparently not rare, because there are several strong warnings. For example, in the "Wisdom learning of Ani": "do not overdo with the beer you drink from a jug. If you talk you will make an incorrect statement from your mouth. If you fall and break your legs, there is no one there who can give you a hand; your drinking companions get up and say: away with the drunk! If someone comes to look for you and to question you, one finds you on the floor, and you are like a small child."

Herodotus reports that at meals of rich people, after the meal, "a man passed around a picture of someone in a coffin; the coffin is identical to the painted counterfeet, cut out

133

and one or two yards long. This is shown to each one at the party and he says: drink and be happy, but look at this, because you will be like it when you are dead. This is the custom at their drinking parties."

In the archives in Brussels there is a teacher's document in which is written to a student, "I heard that you neglect the papyri and devote yourself to dances. You go from the pub to the tavern; beer vapors show your way. People avoid you when you waver through the street . . . ."

Beer was made quite differently from ours: wheat or other cereals were humidified and buried in the earth until they started to ferment. Then it was ground and mixed with yeast to make a dough, formed in loafs which were baked for a short enough period that the insides remained raw. The loaves were then broken and placed in water. The mixture was allowed to ferment for one day. It was then filtered and the beer was ready to drink.

Spiritual and Divine Order

Celebrate a good day,
Place balsam and sweet scent at your nose,
On your breast garlands of lotus and
love apples
While the woman of your heart sits next
to you
Get chants and deliver it to your eyes
Look over everything that is bad and think
of the joys till the day comes,
On which you land in that land,
that loves silence.
(Song of the harpists in the tomb of Neferhotep)

"When there were no people or hunters and there was no death, land and water were formed from the primeval chaos." This is how creation is described in the pyramid. What appears to be creation is explained in the "Divine Teaching from Memphis" regarding the work of the creator god, Ptah. "He created the gods, he made the cities, he founded the regions, he placed the gods in their cult places, he determined the sacrifices, he founded their shrine, he made their body of all types of wood, all types of rocks, all types of clay, and all types of other things that grew on him [Ptah] in which they formed a shape."

These teachings from a creator god were put aside by the theological school of Heliopolis, because the creator god of Heliopolis, Atum, came from the chaotic original water, the Nun. With the passage of time (to about the Twelfth Dynasty),

135

Atum fused with the sun god, Re, to Re-Atum or Amon-Re. He received the honors of kings and achieved state cult.

Re was in the center of all life in ancient Egypt as the origin of life. He swam in the waters of the sky as the sun barge, which went up and down with the disk of the sun. A special poetic statement of faith has been handed to us as the "Sun Song of Amarna" of Pharaoh Akhenaten, who lived around 1360 BC. In a translation by the Egyptologist Kurt Sethe, it reads:

> You appear so lovely in the light region of the sky, you living sun, who started to live first!
> You have started to shine in the place of eastern light and filled all lands with your beauty.
> You are beautiful and big, shining and high over all lands.
> Your rays contain the lands until the end of all those that you created; you are the sun and penetrate for this reason to its outer end.
> You subdue it for your beloved son.
> You are far away still, your rays are on the Earth; you are in the face of mankind, and still your way is not known.
> When you go to rest, in the area of western light the world is dark, as in death.
> The sleepers are in the rooms, the heads covered, no eye can see another.
> All things are stolen, while they lay under their head; they do not notice it.
> Every vermin thing appears from its den, all vermin bites; the darkness is as attractive to them as for others a fire.
> The world lies quiet, since the one who created it went to rest in the area of light.
> In the morning gray you shine again on us and shine anew as the Sun in the day. You

drive away the darkness, as soon as you bestow your rays . . . .

> Your rays penetrate to the inside of the sea.
> You are the one who lets the seed develop in women, you who changes water into people, who maintains the son alive in the body of the mother, who calms him, so that his tears stop. Nurse of the child in the mother's body. You who provide the air to maintain life of all of your creatures.
> When it goes down in the body of the woman, the breath, on the day of the birth you soon open his mouth completely and take care of his needs . . . .
> When you start to glow, you let [every arm] move for the king, and [speed] is in all legs, since you created the world.
> You raise them again for your son, who came out of your body, King Akhenaten and the Queen Nefertiti.

For association between political and religious representations, the Egyptians kept, in addition to the creator god, a large number of local gods. Osiris, for example, was originally only a local great in the eastern delta, as was his sister and wife, Isis, and son, Horus. (Osiris' murder and dismemberment have already been discussed). This myth is found in many interpretations and forms: as war between light and darkness; as comparison of fertile soil and desert; as changing and blooming nature. The Egyptian cult for the dead Osiris establishes, however, the most important connection between people of the living world to the afterlife or other world, as is the most important move in the chess game between the pharaoh and the divinities. Since a god could die, so could the pharaoh.

Since the god kept his power after death, the dead king also kept his power and divinity.

A number of theological statements appear on coffins' and tombs' texts. It is surprising too that the gods could be questioned about the afterlife. From approximately the year 2000 BC comes this "discussion between someone tired of life and his soul":

> When you get to the burial, this is only heart pain. It is only bringing about of tears, and making people cry. It means bringing people from their house and throwing them onto the desert hills. Never will you come up, to see the light of the sun again! Those that construct in granite and make pretty pyramids obtain an imposing work—as soon as builders became god, their sacrificial stones were destroyed as were those of the tired who died on the dike without successors. The water took part, and the heat of the sun did the rest. Only the fish of the land at the margins talked to them. Therefore, hear me! See, it is good, when mankind hears: follow the happy day! Forget the worry....

Already ideas of the end of the world existed. Osiris and Atum, the god of creation, discussed a major catastrophe that Osiris had asked about. Atum says, "You will be longer than millions and millions of years. I will, however, destroy everything I created. The earth will again appear as a creating ocean, as a water flood as at the beginning. I will be all that will remain, together with Osiris, after I have again transformed myself into a serpent, which nobody knows, which does not see any god."

A type of "lower court" seems to have been the Egyptian "death court." Pharaoh Khety (First Intermediate Period) wrote for his son in the "Teachings for Merikare":

> ... the judges that judge the wretched, you know, are not mild, and each day when misery is judged, in that hour, one is at his post. The accuser is bad. Do not play with the smart and do not rely on the length of years, because they see a lifetime as an hour. When the human being is left to die, his deeds are placed in a pile next to him. Eternity, however, guards it, that man is there, and a fool is one who makes a fuss about it. Those, however, who come without having sinned, will be like a god there, walking free like the masters of eternity....

If the sun with all life under it went down, the dead awoke in the afterlife in the kingdom of Osiris. He belongs to the group of the "Great of the New Era." Thoth was the physician of the gods. He is pictured in the official seal of the University of Cairo. The ancient Egyptians believed that when the sun god left the underworld in the morning to wash away the night colors in the Sea Jaru, and then to embark with the reddish appearance in the eastern lit mountains, then he also removed his ram's head, and with his falcon's head walked through awakening nature. Then it is said in a hymn that "he is praised by the baboons."

The god Thoth was represented with a baboon's head on which there was a slice of moon, the emblem of knowledge. Thoth's sacred animal was an ibis. In the endless labyrinths of Hermopolis, over four million jars with ibises were found.

The sphinx, of course, also belongs to the world of animals. The pharaohs placed their head on a lion's body to demonstrate the strength and force of the "king of the animals." The head was covered with a cloth which was decorated with the first serpent, which since the unification of kingdoms was a sign of the ruling of the kings.

The ancient Egyptians were wanderers between worlds: between this and the "other" world, between gods and animals; they were looking for the order of life. They did not see their lives as ending with death, because from the "land of the living," they entered the "house of eternity," where they placed themselves "alive" in peace. Diodore from Sicily wrote: "They consider the time of life very short; the time afterwards, however, very long. Therefore, they call the homes of the living 'here mountains,' the tombs, 'eternal houses.' The time that they spend on Earth is only a dream; one says welcome to the one who arrived in the west."

The "Ka"—the indestructible creation personality—accompanies the dead body into the afterworld, where the transformation to the eternal body occurs. Whatever the person started on Earth, he continued in the afterlife towards completion. The ritual of rebirth is, therefore, in the formula: "Awake, oh the ill, you who are asleep. They lifted your head in the direction of the horizon.

Come! Your head will not be taken from you in the future! Your head will not be taken from you in eternity!"

As early as the pre-dynastic era, the Egyptians tried to save the body after death. Life after departure seemed to ancient Egyptians to be determined by three things: the body, Ka, and Ba. This may seem somewhat confusing to us (and probably was also to the Egyptians). These ideas translate somewhat shakily into our idea of the "soul."

As the ram-headed god, Khnum, created man, he had on his potter's wheel the body and Ka—the divine, living, undying matter. Ba is born from the union of the body and Ka, and is something similar to the conscience. When the body dies, Ka and Ba are united. "He is going to his Ka" was said among the common folk when somebody died. Ka and Ba took responsibility before the gods. The ancient Egyptians believed that Ka could take the human body again at any time to return to its original body. The "vessel" had to be available; therefore, one mummified the cadaver.

Since the body had to "survive" for this, tomb rites became more extreme. From the initially small vaults were devised large rooms and halls with cunningly simulated tombs and pitfalls. There was more food and house material. Gold and jewels were introduced into the tombs so that the body would not want for anything on the long trip. Even from the earliest times the tombs were robbed by thieves, which is why the priests moved from Giza and Saqqara to West Thebes. There the "Valley of the Kings" was constructed as long tunnels in the rock to bury the pharaohs and their wealth. It was to no avail, however, as the thieves cunningly discovered the tombs. Nothing remained untouched—except the tomb of the "forgotten" pharaoh: Tutankhamun, which was opened in this century.

Dreams and astrology

Prophecy and dream interpretation played a major role in ancient Egypt and also in medicine. From the slave to the pharaoh, man submitted to prophecy, for everyday events as well as major campaigns.

The True Egyptian Dream Book, which is also sold today, was available in the following form (the individual prophesies are similar to today's): the person who in a dream sees himself as dead will have a long life; he who dreams that he is losing his teeth knows a relative who will die; and the one who sees himself in the mirror, "this is bad, it means a second woman. Those who dream of a large cat will have a large harvest, he who climbs a mast will lift his god. However, he who dreams that he is eating cucumbers will have a fight. Should he dream that he is eating figs and grapes, he will suffer illness."

The book comes from the New Kingdom, and its form is a simple, easy, "peasant thought pattern." At the time of Herodotus (at least, we can come to this conclusion from his work), prophesying must have swept ancient Egypt like a fever. Immediately Herodotus noticed that the cradle of astrology and alchemy were on the Nile. The original discoveries were still true in later centuries. So, Thoth, the god to whom most knowledge was attributed (also in the Papyrus Ebers), became the Greek's Hermes. During the Middle Ages, the alchemical writings of Hermes Trimegistos (the "three-times great") were organized. For this reason, we still speak of "hermetic works."

According to Herodotus, Egyptians founded astrology, and Aristotle considered Egyptians to be the first astronomers. Each Egyptian hour had its fixed planet which produced luck or sorrow, and the horoscope depended, of course, on the constellations. Amun (Jupiter) always brought luck. Seb (Saturn) brought sorrow, and Thoth (Mercury) brought a merry nature. The different stars also had an influence on the different members.

Champollion also occupied himself with the works *(Letters, p. 23a Firmicus Maternus IV, 16)* of astrology and astronomy. "The monuments are probably of astronomical disposition, and the ceremonial calendar which came to us confirms what the classicists say about the astronomy of the Egyptians." The names of two famous astrologers should not be omitted: they are Petrosiris and Nechepso.

The Book of
the Dead

My Pharaoh

I wished that the end of humanity
was here
that there could be no more conception
and no more birth.
If only the noise of the land would stop
and there would be no more fighting.

Death stands before me
as if a sick one
gets well, as if one
after an illness, goes out.
Death stands before me
like the smell of myrrh,
as if one
on a windy day
sits under the sail.
Death stands before me
like the smell of lotus blossoms,
as if one
sits drunk
on the shore.
Death stands before me
like a worn path,
as if one
comes home from the war.
Death stands before me
like a clear sky,
as one comes to that
which he does not know.

Death stands before me
as if someone longs
to see his house again,
after he has spent
many years in prison.
(Song of Ipuwer)

Before we treat mummification as the last chapter of the medicine of the pharaohs, it is important to describe the culture in which the idea of preparing a body for eternity formed. Time and death were essential ideas for the philosophy of the Egyptians. It was a station of the long journey without beginning or end. Death initiated the birth of eternal life; a birth on Earth was obviously a death in the afterworld, thus it was an eternal circle. Or, as the Greek philosopher Heraklitus of Ephesus said so well, "Immortals: mortal mortals: immortals, because the life of these is the death of the others, and the life of others is the death of these."

The French historian Albert Champdor, in his work on the Egyptian *Book of the Dead* wrote:

We cannot imagine how this unification [of ancient Egypt] with the world could take place, and while we are not able to separate ourselves from the present, and in our most secret person let us be conquered by Ka.... Today we are happy to embark on such abstract ways because they are apparently not based on anything substantial that we do not know, that cannot be seen, and continues to develop or else perishes without this development or destruction entering our understanding or feeling in any way. Our unseen being exists in spite of it. Our being is, because of this indestructible and immortal...this double picture of ourselves is what awakens the Egyptian to life. For all dead of all previous and future eras, *his* being as long as eternity awaits...and all dead will rise again as each morning the sun comes up—the bringer and giver of endless life energy.

Then, what is the Egyptian *Book of the Dead*? It is a book of prayers, a collection of sayings of the scribes Hunefer, Ani, and the Amun-priestess, AnHai, which was placed in the tombs with the dead either in the coffin or wrapped with the mummy bandages. The *Book of the Dead* is composed of about 200 chapters of various lengths. With it, a dead person should be able to find his way back in the underworld ("Duat") where he had twelve regions to cross (discussed later). During the burial ceremonies, the priestess recited these "prayers."

The papyri with the death sayings are again attributed to Thoth, the god of the scribes. They were probably written during the New Kingdom. The name comes from the German Egyptologist Karl Richard Lepsius (1810–1884). He established the Egyptian Museum in Berlin and also undertook the division of the *Book of the Dead* into chapters. His Swiss pupil, Edouard Henri Naville, in 1886 placed all the known sayings (1,844 in number) into one work. The *Book of the Dead* was also known as the *Book of the Sun Litanies, Book of the Gates, Book of the Hidden Residence, Book of the Breathing,* or *Book from that which is in the Duat.* The best example of a collection of a text is from the seventh century BC and is held in the Egyptian Museum in Turin.

One of the repeated pictures on the Egyptian tomb walls (papyrus copies of which can be bought in all tourist centers today) is the famous scene of weighing the soul of the dead. The gods are sitting in trial and hearing the testimonial of faith of the dead one. His heart (his conscience) is weighed. If the balance tips to the right side, that is the feather of Maat, then Amenuit (the devourer of the souls) does not interfere. Instead the dead one is conducted by Horus to the divine guardian of the pillars, and Anubis will then say that a new righteous one has been born in the face of Osiris.

Before Thoth and the jackal-headed Anubis, the dead one must explain that he:

Did not commit any sin against the people; has not done anything of which the gods may not approve; respected the hierarchies; did not kill anyone or order anyone to be killed; did not inflict pain; was never stingy when, without witnesses, he measured food and wine that were to be presented in sacrifices in the temple; that he did not remove the food and drink from the dead; that he did no wrong in the areas of cleanliness; did not shorten the yard to take away land from his neighbor; did not falsify measurements and weights; neither removed the birds of the gods nor the fish from the sacred seas; did not injure the herds of the Thebes of Amun; and did not wrongly weigh the gold bars intended for the treasury of the gods.

The dead one has to present himself before the gods and say:

I used life to bring good; without lies, O eternal and well-disposed gods, I can sing my song of praise, since I have the best conscience in front of the gods. I gave food to those who needed it, and water to those who were thirsty in the middle of the day; my fishing boat I loaned to those who had none. I did not sin in Heliopolis! The carriers of the flames of Kher-Aha, I did not cheat! For the swallowing of the shadows, I did not kill anyone! For the double sky lionesses, I did not steal any corn! For the destroyer of the dead remains of Heracleopolis, I did not plunder the temple wealth! I wrapped my parents in a dead cloth. I did not send the daughter of my servant into slavery. The vultures of the skies I revered since they are sacred animals. Not once as long as I live, was I tried by the magistrate, or did I make a sign that he should frighten the soul of a dead one, a sign that would have given a picture of unclean things *(According to a translation by Jean Capart).*

Then the dead one arrives at the steps of praise of the West End:

Praise to thee, O gods, who recognize the smell of those that come from the soil of Egypt and appear before you, after embalming, wrapped in cloth and covered with magic unguents, that allowed the division and brought out the inner being from the outer one, when it was permitted, as was once the case of Phoenix of Heracleopolis, which is the soul of Re. Praise to thee, O Gods in Osiris swaddling cloths, who are behind the gates of Amenti and know how to recognize those whose limbs are decaying and stink, because they killed their equals, or stole the animals in the temple, or were impure in seclusion, or dirtied the water of the river. Praise to thee, in eternity, divine souls, souls with the baboon's head! I who am dead, and reborn, I have made sure before I came in front of you that my dead body would be washed and swaddled in cloth, and my eyes painted with antimony. I know that I did not break the developing egg, nor did I swear at the goat of Mendes, nor did I say the name of Ptah-Tatenem in Abydos. Save me! Protect me with your closeness, because my breath is clean, my heart is clean, my hands are clean, and those that see me say: welcome, you who are clean, and may your soul have peace in the underworld.... Be welcome, because you have cleaned your bowels in the sea of Maat, and you can appear—you, who are clean—in front of Osiris, the steer of Amenti, before Osiris Neberdjer, before Osiris Djedi, whose spinal column is the axis of the world.

The following describes how the Egyptians imagined the kingdom of the dead. A bright strip of fruitful land was divided by a river. And this underworld had—as did the upper world—twelve regions, called the Duat. They were divided by powerful gates (therefore also the name *Book of the Gates*) which contained terrible monsters. The clean souls who knew the cleansing sayings could travel with Re in the sun boat through the regions during the night, and shine with him in the morning, and travel another night in the boat through the Duat on a rope that was a living boa.

With the sun boat through the Duat

Here is the description of the twelve-hour voyage through the twelve Duat of the underworld from the *Book of the Dead:*

In the first hour of the *Book of the Dead,* the first hour of the night, the dead notice, filled with fear of the dragon that guards the entrance to hell and spits fire. When the dead are smart, they carry protective amulets, and if they know magic formulas, they will be able to elude the awareness of the terrible Cerberus of the underworld and continue through the twisting of the fearful way. So they go through the gate of the west in the first region to the other side. In the second and third hour the dead pass through the Anrutef gate, the gate of the kingdom of the souls, and discover the cold zones, in the regions of Uernes and Osiris. They greet the ram-headed sun which came from the west, the boundary between the kingdom of the living for those who still have living breath and a white skin, not a green one. The dead demonstrate respect to the sun, which became their corpse, their flesh, as they left the boat of the day to take the barge of the night to make the journey through the twelve regions of the underworld, before they rise again under the eye of the Sphinx, as they have done every day since the beginning of time. *[For your information: the Sphinx in Giza with the head of Pharaoh Khephren is placed in such a manner that in the morning his eyes look precisely at the sun when it comes up on the horizon.]*

In the fourth and fifth hour the judges watch as the sun passes through the secret passages of Sokaris, the old god of the dead with the face of a falcon from the region of Memphis. The darkness is there like the water in the deep of the sea and Re will not look again at those that stay there. In the meantime, the dead, who are clammy as mud, can hear his voice while he gives orders. The sacred barge will then continue its way through the darkness of Sokaris and will transform itself into a long serpent, which in this terrible, hellish night will be almost invisible.

In the sixth hour the dead will see thousands of souls of birds and foreign goddesses who carry the pupils of the eyes of Horus in their hands. They will see Khepre, the scarab, and five-headed dragons armed with daggers. In the seventh hour the dead will stay before Isis, who has a righteous wrath against the demons. They see the enemies of Osiris, who were beheaded by lion-headed gods and chained like Asiatics. They see the back side of the terrestrial firmament and the Apophis serpent which fills the seventh circle of hell with its slimy coils and drinks away the water under the sun barge in order to delay its journey. In the eighth hour the dead will be happy for the noise of the "meowing" of the risen who are coming out from their houses under the Earth to greet the sun and to praise its sunshine again.

In the night until the eleventh hour the dead cross the water and the fire of all the hellish world that is named in the text, Agarit. The oarsmen now leave the sun barge and return to their secret hells. The rope that was used in pushing the barge through its night course transforms itself into a serpent, and a scarab sits down next to the sun.

In the twelfth and last hour, the dead finally see the sun which, before it will shine again in the world of the living, will be born again in the form of a scarab. Nut will deliver every new sun that will appear between her thighs and make it come out from her genitals. Let the dead rejoice and the living rise to look at the light; because from the lap of Hell the dead sun came again to Kheorem, the god of the morning sun, to the new god, who after so much misery and metamorphosis in the twelve regions in the underworld was reborn again.

From below, however, one hears noises when the noise of the people subsides....

Moreover, the litanies of the *Book of the Dead* were not recited only at funerals of people. The priests also said them on mummification of cats and falcons, rats and toads, serpents and crocodiles. The ceremony was the same, as if it were the funeral of a pharaoh. At Hermopolis, an enormous hall cut into the rock was found in which sacred ibises were embalmed and mummified after the prayers of the *Book of the Dead* had been recited. The archaeologist Cabra (as described in Champdor's *Das Ägyptische Totenbuch*) discovered the "labyrinth of uncountable ways and halls. In one hall in which there was an altar, we discovered a sitting baboon and two ibises cut in wood and covered with gold. All three animals looked at the door, behind which was the tomb of the high priest, Ankhor. Vases of alabaster and 365 statues of shining faience were used in the cult of the dead. Our surprise was boundless in seeing such an ibis cult, such an enormous palace under the earth."

The Trip to the Other Side

*O you who can make the wings of time
strike faster, you inhabitant of all
secrets of life,
you guard of all words I say—see, you are
ashamed of mine, your son,
your heart is full of sorrow, full of shame
whether my heavy sins in this world,
whether my malice and lapses.
O, make peace with me, make peace,
remove the divisions that part us!
Let all my sins be washed away,
so that they can be forgotten.
They fall on your right and your left.
Yes, remove all of my badness,
remove the mud that fills your heart,
so that we can have peace in the future.*
(From the Book of the Dead*)*

The biggest mystery of Egypt—the embalming of the dead—opens to us another remarkable view of the ancient Egyptian medical world. Careful calculations indicate that 500 million bodies were mummified up until the time of the Romans! At the beginning of the Middle Kingdom, the seat of power shifted from Memphis to Thebes, and on the western shore of the Nile—on the other side of the legendary political and religious center—real mummification factories must have developed. In the times of the Fourth Dynasty, mummification was a right of the pharaohs. During the following centuries, people of the "better classes" were also mummified, and by the time of the

Persian domination, just about every-one—whether peasant or sculptor—was mummified.

Let us again turn to Herodotus, for a detailed account of mummification:

When in a house in Egypt a person, naturally someone who has some worth, dies, all women in the house cover their heads, including the face, with clay; then they let the dead one remain in the house while they run through the city, exalted with bare chest, and beat themselves and all other female relatives on the chest. The men also will strike themselves as a sign of sorrow and they too are exalted. When this has taken place, they take the body for embalming.

For this there are special persons who understand the art. When they get the body, they show to the relatives samples of body configurations in wood and those painted close to reality, and tell them the best manner of embalming—names of which I am too shy to use. Then they show them the second [cheaper] and finally the third [least expensive] one. They ask in which manner the body is to be treated. The relatives bargain about the price and leave. However, they keep the corpse in the house with them.

This is the way of the careful and expensive art of embalming. First they remove the brain with a bent iron through the nostrils in the following way: in part they remove it, in part they place medicines in it. Then they open the abdominal region with a sharp stone knife and remove all the internal organs. They clean them, wash them with palm wine, and cover them with pulverized incense. They then fill the abdominal cavity with pure pulverized myrrh with cassia leaves and other perfumes mixed with incense and close the corpse again. The corpse is then placed in salt for seventy days; one cannot leave them longer than that. When the seventy days have passed,

they wash the corpse and cover the whole body with bandages of fine byssus cloth and coated with rubber which the Egyptians frequently use instead of glue. Then the relatives take the corpse and make a coffin of wood in the form of a person, place the corpse inside, and take it to the tomb chamber, where they place the corpse against the wall.

They thus take good care of the corpses that have been embalmed for the most expensive price. However, when the relatives select the intermediate form to avoid the high costs, the following is done to the corpses: they introduce enemas of cedar oil and fill the lower abdomen of the dead without opening or removing the stomach and the internal organs. They inject it from the bottom in such a manner that the enema is not expelled and then place the corpse for the prescribed seventy days in sodium carbonate. On the last day they remove the cedar oil, which has such an effect that the stomach and the internal organs come out with it. The flesh, however, is dissolved by the sodium carbonate so that the only remaining parts of the corpse are the skin and the bones. The corpse at this time is returned to the relatives, and nothing else is done to it.

The third form of embalming, used by those with the least amount of means, is as follows: the abdominal cavity is cleaned with purgative oils and salts . . . for seventy days, and then the corpse is returned to the family.

When the wives of important men, or those who are very pretty or important, die, they are not given immediately to the embalmers. Only after three or four days are they given to the embalmers. This is done to prevent the embalmers from practicing any lewdness on the women. Because someone was discovered who was doing lewd acts with a fresh female corpse, and it was denounced . . . .

It is not known who in the

early days of Egyptian history "discovered" the technique of embalming. Someone probably experimented with animals and the corpses of slaves and captives, and in the beginning the dead were only buried in hot sand, since they would dehydrate in this manner. This was obviously not sufficient since they started placing the corpses in wooden coffins. After the drying method with sodium carbonate was found, and the need for removal of the soft tissues of the abdomen and skull was recognized, the priests and the embalmers kept the technique to themselves for thousands of years.

Mummies have been found dating from the year 3400 BC. One of the oldest is the mummy of the mother of Pharaoh Khufu (Cheops). In the Old Kingdom, the methods of mummification were not perfect. The abdominal cavity was still filled with cloth, and some bodies were broken into pieces. Petrie believed that the bodies were damaged during the process of tissue removal, but this is questioned by the mummy researcher Elliot Smith. According to Smith, tomb thieves broke the mummies to steal their jewels. Religious Egyptians later (however incorrectly) re-pieced them together.

With the passage of time, the technique of mummification became perfected. The high point came during the New Kingdom. Tutankhamun, the young pharaoh, was wrapped in sixteen long pieces of linen and placed in three coffins of gold, a fourth one of stone, and then three more of wood.

Until the beginning of the New Kingdom (about 1550 BC), the heart was left in place and only the viscera and blood vessels were removed from the body. During the New Kingdom, often the heart was removed as well. This was done for fear of the dead tribunal; it was feared that one's own heart could betray one and say negative things. In other times, the muscles of the arms and legs were removed and the skin filled with resin-impregnated papyrus. The removed organs, which had been cleaned, were filled with myrrh and sodium carbonate mixed in a special type of urn, the so-called Kanope, which was placed with the mummy in the tomb.

Each pharaoh had his own embalming temple. The common mortal was "treated" in a tent or a cloth pavilion. The roof could easily be removed and the pavilion could be constructed again somewhere else, according to need. The temple or the tent was called "uabit," the "clean place."

The main persons in necropolis were, of course, the embalmers. After all, without them there was no "afterlife" of the body and with this the immortality of Ka. A large group of specialists worked with them. The first was the "parashiste," the cutter. He had the task of opening the body and removing the viscera and organs. He then let his colleague, the "taricheute," work on the corpse. He had to care for the conservation of the body; the Greek word for this was, however, also used in fish factories: "salter." The Greek term "chereb" is considerably more poetic; it means the "reader," because texts were read during the embalming ritual. It is possible that at different times these two activities were performed by the same person.

The embalmers were surrounded by a number of assistants and priests; all of the priests wore the mask of Anubis, symbol of the jackal-headed god who had already supervised the embalming of Osiris. The office of embalmer was hereditary and certainly lucrative. However, this profession was not highly regarded. In the Papyrus Sallier III it is said, "the fingers of the embalmer bring badness, they smell of corpses. His eyes burn from heat. He is too tired to read to his own daughter. He spends his days with the cutting of rags because clothing is for him an abomination."

As soon as the corpse was delivered to the embalmer, he started with the removal of the brain. The brain was unimportant to the Egyptians, since the seat of understanding was considered to be in the heart. With long bronze sticks, on which there were spirals and hooks, the brain was removed through the nostrils, piece by piece—tiring work, where it was not always possible to avoid breaking one of the nasal conchae.

There were, however, more radical methods. For King Ahmose,

the head was cut off and the brain spooned out from the skull. Afterwards, the head was placed on a stick, united with the body, and bandaged to it. In another method, one eye was removed and pushed into the brain. We also know of skulls that were opened in the neck region, and after removal of the brain mass, closed again. Also, the brain was not removed in all mummies. At the time of the First Dynasty this was not at all usual, while during Greek times it was done in about fifty percent of all mummifications.

After the brain was removed, the embalmer removed the intestines from the corpse. This was done with a stone knife that the embalmer had made, using a sharp cut from the last rib to the pubic hair. After the reign of Tuthmosis II, the cut was in the groin. First, the embalmer removed the intestines from the body, rolled them up and cut them into several pieces. After that, he removed the spleen, liver, stomach, gallbladder, and often the kidneys too. The bladder was usually left alone. In some mummies, the testicles and the penis were amputated and were handled separately, we do not know why. Then the embalmer entered the chest cavity through the diaphragm, cut the trachea and esophagus and removed the lungs. The heart remained in place. If it was cut along with the lungs, it was placed back into the body and sometimes even sutured there.

Now came the complicated

activity of drying the body, since humans are seventy-five percent water. After much guessing and many arguments, scientists have agreed that the drying was performed with sodium carbonate—not with hot sand, or fires, or with salt—because one found sodium carbonate-covered embalming sticks and sodium carbonate crystals in the mummies. One question remains: was it liquid or dried sodium carbonate? Lucas, a chemist of the eighteenth century, did experiments in this area. He placed an eviscerated pigeon in salt solution, in three percent sodium carbonate solution, and in dry sodium carbonate; a fourth one he placed in grainy salt. After forty days, he removed the birds from the sodium carbonate and the salt. The pigeons from the sodium carbonate were in good condition, he only had to wash them and let them dry in the sun. Those that were in the salt solution were a mass of skin, bones, and fat without form. The salt and sodium carbonate pigeons, however, were hard and firm, jut as we know the mummies. In this manner it was demonstrated that the ancient Egyptians used dry sodium carbonate for dehydration of the body.

After a thorough washing, the mummy was stuffed with different items that range from sawdust, to cloth remnants, to clay jugs. For the most part, the body looked real. It was important that before bandaging it be well dried. That this was not always the case is demonstrated by the mold found in some mummies.

The dried body had to be improved with the use of unguents. In the Papyrus Boulaq 3 it is described in the following manner: "First, head creams with incense resin; perfume the body with the exception of the head; prepare the back with an oil massage. Second, rub the head and bandages of the body. Last, head rubbing and rubbing of the hands and feet."

The main ingredients of the oils and creams were cedar oil, caraway seed oil, wax, raw rubber, turpentine oil, incense, and sodium carbonate.

Before closing the body, a coating of resin had to be placed on each angle. This was very expensive because in Egypt there were no pine trees, so the resin had to come from Syria. History tells us that Alexander the Great was preserved in honey. If this is correct, this certainly did not happen often, despite a story from Giza that during an excavation a jar with honey was found that was still usable. The honey was removed and the corpse of a child was found, completely dressed and in perfect condition.

After the resin and filling, the corpse was once more corrected for skin, nails, and eyes. The bandaging of the corpse was done under the supervision of a chief embalmer. He also wore a jackal mask and said the litanies corresponding to the rites for the complicated and lengthy performances. Between the bandages, amulets were placed, for example Djed-pillars, isis blood, udjat-eyes, scarabs of gold, bronze, stone, glass, faience, or clay.

The complexity of placing the bandages is described in the ninth chapter of the *Ritual of Embalming:*

So we start with the embalming of the god, and bandage his left hand, which has been rubbed with the same oil. Place in it "Anch-imy," a plant, bitumen from Coptos, one part, and sodium carbonate one part in the first. Wrap his ... with a cloth strip of royal linen, followed by a bandage. Put the gold signet ring on his finger and gild his closed fist again after it has acquired the correct position by placement of a tampon of cloth. Cover the back of the right hand to the base of the fingers with oil, make thirty-six packages of "Anch-imy" plants, sodium carbonate, bitumen, and the "senebnetjeri" plant, finish the tie and place the hand close to the left hand. Tie "mensa" plant and a branch of "aru" tree with a "senebnetjeri" plant together in his left hand and think that he is the "aru" tree Osiris. Place a piece of cloth over which was poured "aru" resin so that everything stays in position in the hand. On this cloth there must be the picture of Hapi, the greatest of all gods, because with this cloth the re-born will dress himself. On a cloth tampon rolled up six times there should be a picture of Isis in pure smoke yellow. ... Now place the cloth of Isis from Coptos over the hand, after you have first pressed those of Hapi and Isis in it. They shall never be separated from him. Bandage the hand tightly over the cloth.

Before the mummy was given to the "House of Eternity," the ritual of the "mouth opening" was performed. The embalmed person should symbolically come alive again and his soul and body vigor; the Ka and the Ba, in this manner, have the possibility of returning to the body. This ritual also took place on the statue of the dead which was also considered by the Egyptians to be a living creature.

An old description of the ceremony says:

One opened the mouth of the statue with several tools, tongs (both named by the gods) and a type of cross-hatchet (great in magic). At this moment, the son he loved appeared, a name that of course reminds us of Horus in the Osiris mysteries. One opened the mouth again with a chisel and a gold finger. Then, one offered the sculpture of the dead a cover for the head, a knife with a manlike head at the end, grapes, an ostrich feather, and a cup filled with water. Again slaughter, again sacrifices were made, and the dead was offered the heart and leg of the animal. After a new mouth opening with the cross-hatchet and an associated incense offering, the dead received a series of sacrifices for his protection .... Now the rubbing with salves started, after which the statue was made up, scepter and club were removed, incense brought. A drink offering made the sacrifice ceremony final.

With the progressing decadence of the Egyptian kingdom, there was also a deterioration of the quality of mummification. Also, religious feelings changed. Mummies from the Twenty-first Dynasty are completely neglected, lovelessly put together, sometimes without a head or without arms, or with legs that originally did not belong to those corpses. On a tomb of the late era in Tuna el-Gebel are the words:

I am the son of Epimachus. Do not pass by my grave indifferently. Your nose will not be bothered by the unpleasant smell of cedar oil [remember Herodotus' description of the second-class funeral with the enema-oil; it was not cedar oil but juniper The wood was distilled and mixed with turpentine oil and tar, which produced a corroding acid.] Lend your ear a little to a good-smelling dead person. Death came for me with a cough and I died, as all men have to die. So do not cry my friend, I hate tears. I also asked my cousin, Philermos, to dismiss all complaints, and not to bury me, only to dig me out. Bury me only once and without cedar oil. The long burial rites, the crying women do not make me happy, because all men must die.

Perhaps this boy, who died at the age of twelve—probably of tuberculosis—was cremated. In Roman times that was usual. Eventually one did not remove the viscera from the corpse; one covered the dead only with salt or sodium carbonate, left it in normal dress, and buried it.

What the mummies tell us

In the year 1859 a certain Marc Armand Ruffer was born in Lyon. By chance, he went to England where he studied medicine. After returning to Paris, Ruffer decided to dedicate himself to bacteriology. During the course of his research, he suffered an attack of diphtheria from which he had great difficulty recovering. At the age of 34 in 1893 he left for the climate of Cairo, where he be-

came professor of bacteriology at the university. At the same time, Ruffer developed a love for Egyptology, in which his medical knowledge was of great usefulness in his research about mummies. His studies and publications—on over 4,000 old parasites in the mummies or the consequences of incestuous behavior in the pharaonic kingdom—are still valid today. Ruffer, while director of the Red Cross, died in 1917 aboard a boat that was torpedoed at Salonica. The British duo Elliot Smith and F. Wood continued his work (Smith in a very unorthodox manner). About these two the story is still told, with a smile, of how Smith drove through Cairo with the mummy of Pharaoh Tuthmosis III in the passenger seat, in search of an x-ray machine to radiograph the king.

They did not learn much more from the results of these special methods, with which the mummies were and still are studied, and from the remarkable insights into the illnesses of the pharaohs gained from them. The latest examination took place in the Spring of 1990 at Brigham Hospital in Boston, Massachusetts. The radiologist Myron Marx examined eleven coffins from the Museum of Fine Arts with a computer tomography machine, an instrument that is normally used to study tumors and inflammations in loco. The two most imposing coffins contained the remains of the singer Ta-Bes, and her husband, Nes-Ptah, a rich barber. They lived until 950 BC in Thebes. Marx examined them for four hours and then gave his diagnosis. The singer had several rib fractures and a brain tumor. The man, who must have been about sixty, must have been very ill. In addition to major dental problems and a significant positional change of the lumbar vertebra, Marx diagnosed arterial calcification. Since the veins of the legs also had sclerotic plaques down to the heels, the radiologist speculated that the Egyptian could have been diabetic.

In the so called "Münchner Mummy Project" of two years duration, a 2,700-year-old mummy was the middle point of a project funded by the German Republic. A large number of researchers, among them radiologists, anthropologists, and Egyptologists, examined a well-preserved mummy, which had the name "Si Chonsu" on the top of the sarcophagus, at the institute for anthropology and human genetics of the university. This name, however, was not the name of the dead person. It was "Djehuti Irdis," who was found somewhere in the 170-meter-long wrappings, and who had been placed in a stranger's coffin. In unwrapping the external, unimpressive mummy package, the name appeared, then gold-covered nails, and jewel hoops on the arms and legs. The dead person had cloth sandals and a painted cloth on the excellently preserved face. Computer tomography showed that Djehuti died at about age seventeen of tuberculosis. He had blood group A and was 154 centimeters tall.

Early autopsies on mum-mies were not so sophisticated. Egyptologists could only rely on their eyes. On June 1, 1886 Gaston Camille Charles Maspero (who was director general of the Cairo Antiquities Service until 1914) examined the mummy of Ramses II. He noted:

The first cloth layer was removed, and there continued to come cloth strips, about twenty centimeters in width, which were wrapped over the whole body. After this there was another funeral cloth that was stitched together and held together at intervals with thin strips. Then came two long bandages and one piece of fine linen that covered the body from head to toe, and which had about a one-meter drawing of a picture of the goddess, Nut, in red and black, as ritual demanded. Under this amulet there were new wrappings, after that a new layer of four-way folded cloth which was bathed in bitumen. As this last layer was removed, there was Ramses II. He is big (1.72 meters after embalming), of perfect symmetry and well preserved. His long head is small in relation to the body, the upper half head completely bald. His hair is thin at the sides, thicker in the neck, and falls in five-centimeter-long curls to the shoulders. He was white when he died but due to the resins acquired a yellow color. The forehead is low and straight, the eyebrows prominent, the eyelashes white and thick, the eyes are small and placed close to the nose, the nose is long and thin, similar to the hooked Roman nose and is pressed down slightly at the tip from the bandages. The temples are depressed, the cheekbones prominent. The ears are round and stick out but are fine and perforated for the use of earrings like those of a woman; a prominent lower jaw and a high chin. His mouth is wide open and filled by a blackish ointment. Full lips. A small chisel has brought to light some not-so-sharp teeth, which even if very white were very brittle. The thin beard and moustache, probably well barbered during lifetime, grew during illness or after death, the hair is white as the hair on the head and eyelashes, but rough and prickly and at the most, about three to four millimeters long. His skin is a dirty yellow with black spots. His mask gave us some idea how his face must have looked. I would not say it was of great intelligence, possibly a little coarse, however filled with the pride of a royal majesty. Also, the rest of the body is well preserved, only that he does not look so well, his flesh is shrunk, his neck, for example, is not thicker than his spine. The chest is large, the shoulders high, the arms crossed over his chest, his long fine hands are colored with henna, his well-groomed short nails are as well cared for as those of a woman. A wound gapes in his groin from which his viscera were removed. His genitals have been removed by a sharp knife, and have probably been placed, according to custom, in a small wooden statue of Osiris. Thighs and lower legs do not have flesh, the feet are long, thin, a little flat and, like the hands, colored with henna. The bones are black and brittle, the muscles slack through senility and old age. As we know, Ramses II ruled for a while together with his father, Sethos I, and afterwards by himself for sixty-two years. He must have been close to a hundred years old when he died.

For the year 1886 this is certainly a famous work and a very precise examination. However, what science has done in the following 100 years would probably make Maspero cry with envy today.

The next important text was written by Sir Flinders Petrie in the year 1898. Only three years after Wilhelm Conrad Röntgen made his sensational discovery of roentgen rays, Petrie tried roentgen rays on a mummy. The results were still modest. Many followed his idea: Smith and Jones, Bertolotti and Moodie, Jonckheeres and Gray, Harris and Weeks.

In 1900, the method of blood grouping was discovered. Blood determination is also possible with a muscle or a bone that has been reduced to dust. The study of some mummies showed that in ancient Egypt there were blood groups A, B, and O, thus contradicting the supposition that blood group B was a mutation of group O that only took place at the time of Christianity. The study of blood groups of the pharaohs allows us to be certain today that the mummy, for a long time, was considered to be that of Akhenaten and in reality was that of his co-regent, Smenkhkare. For a long time experts discussed whether Smenkhkare and Tutankhamun were brothers. After the blood study, there is nothing to rule it out. They have the same blood factors and are of blood group A2.

Finally, with modern scientific methods there is not much of a problem calculating the age of a mummy. We are no longer dependent on accessories in tombs, types of bandages, and forms of coffins. The radiocarbon method is trustworthy. Put simply, all organic tissues contain carbon 14, which is slightly radioactive. However, each radioactive substance loses radioactivity over time. The time it takes for a material to lose half of its radioactiviy is called its half-life. For carbon 14, the half-life is

5,568 years. Dead tissues do not accumulate new carbon 14. One needs, therefore, only to measure the radioactivity and from it determine the age of the tissue. This takes place by burning the tissue, filtering the carbon from the gas, and measuring with a Geiger counter.

Another method of dating uses the reaction of amino acids and their separation from polarized light.

That almost all mummies have bad teeth has already been discussed; they had caries—probably due to the minerals in the flour of bread. But from what else did the ancient Egyptians suffer? The mummies tell us.

As early as 1909, Ruffer found in the kidneys of two mummies from the Twentieth Dynasty calcified eggs of the worms of bilharziosis; in one mummy from the year 1200 BC he found spores of "black leaves" of pox, and in the lungs and liver of other mummies he found "rod-shaped bacteria, I think, Pest bacilli." In 1910 he examined a mummy of the priest Nesper-e-hap (1000 BC) who had Pott's disease (Percival Pott described it about 1779), tuberculosis of the spinal column, and an abscess in a loin muscle.

Kidney diseases were frequent during the pharaohs' time. Shrunken kidneys and kidney stones too have been recognized for centuries. Today they are considered a consequence of the stress of life in the twentieth century with its gigantic technology, speed, unrest, and poor nutrition, as well as cigarettes and alcohol in an unstable climate. The ancient Egyptian, however, did not let himself be harassed, the climate was relatively constant, hard liquor and tobacco were unknown to him, and in general he lived quite well without fatty meats but with a lot of vegetables, onions, and radishes. In spite of this, he had heart infarcts and suffered from arteriosclerosis. In the mummy found in Deir el-Bahari by Teje, which was that of the wife of Amenophis III, during autopsies the "scar" of an infarct was found. The Parisian physician and medical historian Ange-Pierre Leca, a qualified mummy expert, wrote:

Roentgen pictures often show a calcification of the arteries in the tissues of the limbs. Merenptah, who is usually considered as the pharaoh referred to during the Exodus, and who is supposed to have drowned in the Red Sea, appears on examination not to have died in this manner. He belongs to the first mummies who had a complete anatomical examination and this demonstrated that his aorta has many calcified arteriosclerotic plaques, and not only large arteries, but also in the small capillaries. In the organ packages of the singer Har-Mose of the Eighteenth Dynasty, proof of hardened arteries was found in the form of damaged abdominal arteries. Finally, it is demonstrated that Teje not only suffered from a diseased heart but had high blood pressure. This diagnosis was not delivered by a contemporary physician, but the disease left its unmistakable marks on the kidneys.

The Papyrus Ebers has twenty-one remedies for a cough. The

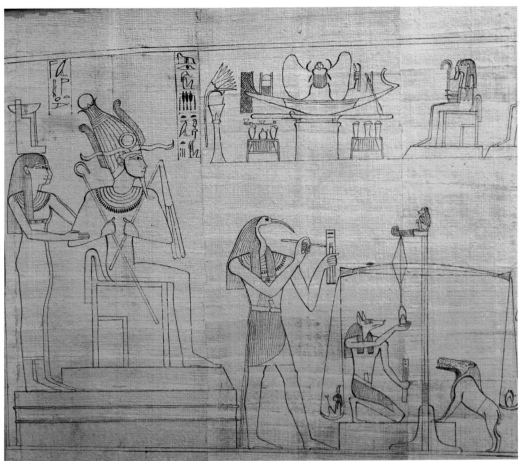

Everyone was scared of this jury in ancient Egypt: a motif from the *Book of Dead of Ani* (Nineteenth Dynasty). The heart of the dead is weighed in the scale of "Maat." Osiris is witness at this jury, the ibis of Thoth writes the "sins" of the sacrifice. If the mistakes of the dead do not rest at least at equilibrium, the heart is eaten by the dog. *British Museum, London.*

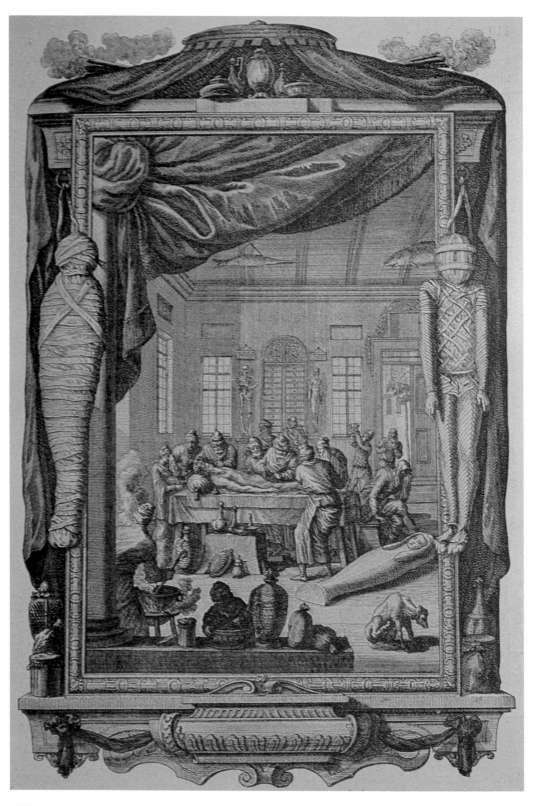

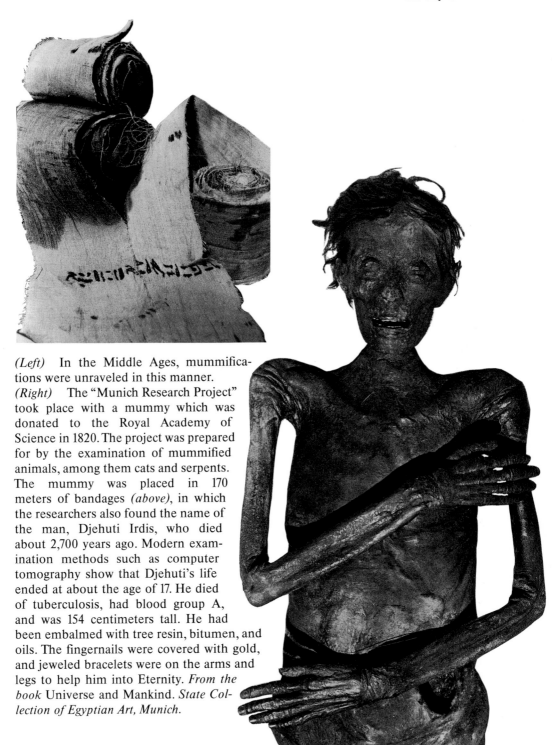

(Left) In the Middle Ages, mummifications were unraveled in this manner.

(Right) The "Munich Research Project" took place with a mummy which was donated to the Royal Academy of Science in 1820. The project was prepared for by the examination of mummified animals, among them cats and serpents. The mummy was placed in 170 meters of bandages *(above)*, in which the researchers also found the name of the man, Djehuti Irdis, who died about 2,700 years ago. Modern examination methods such as computer tomography show that Djehuti's life ended at about the age of 17. He died of tuberculosis, had blood group A, and was 154 centimeters tall. He had been embalmed with tree resin, bitumen, and oils. The fingernails were covered with gold, and jeweled bracelets were on the arms and legs to help him into Eternity. *From the book* Universe and Mankind. *State Collection of Egyptian Art, Munich.*

159

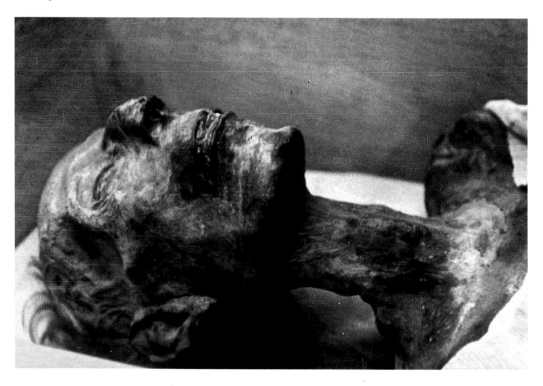

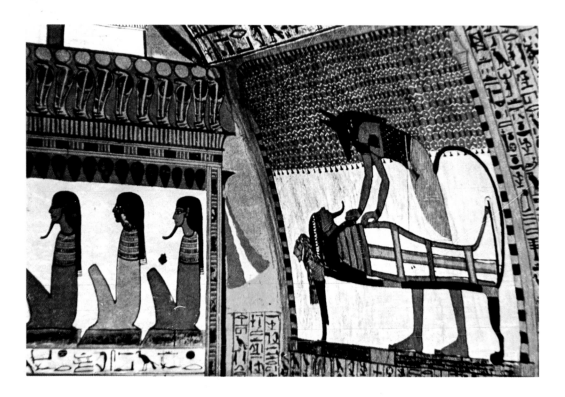

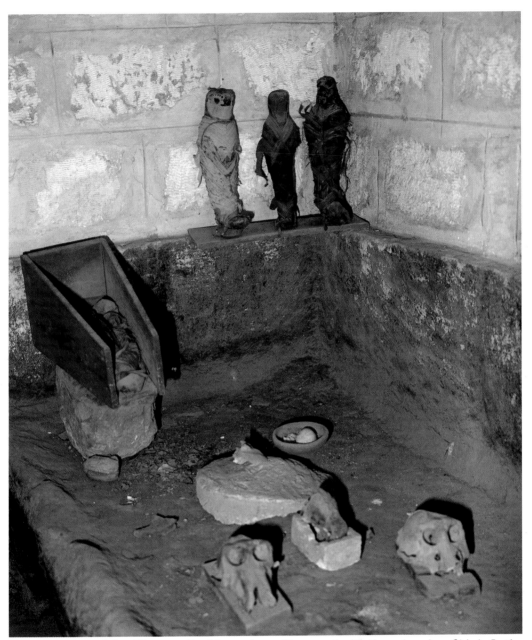

In the suburb of Cairo, Hermopolis, this crypt was discovered with the mummies of birds. In the area around Memphis there are tombs with hundreds of thousands of mummified animals, ibises in particular. Formally one trained by mummifying animals—possibly also slaves—before one dared to work on humans. *Tuna el-Gebel, Hermopolis.*

Opposite page: (Above) The mummy of probably the most remarkable pharaoh of Egypt, Ramses II. No other pharaoh created such monumental tombs and temples, or had more children, or grew to be as old. *Egyptian Museum, Cairo.*
(Below) Anubis the jackal-headed god, symbolized at the mummification of a corpse. *Chapel of Sennutem, Tombs of the Nobles, Thebes.*

161

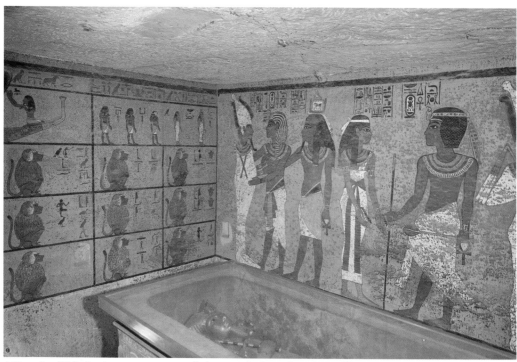

(Above) This is the appearance of the small, hot chamber of Tutankhamun. In the smallest tomb chamber of a pharaoh, unbelievable treasures were found. One of the gold masks is still in place. *Valley of the Kings, Luxor.*

(Below) Extracts from the *Book of the Dead. British Museum, London.*

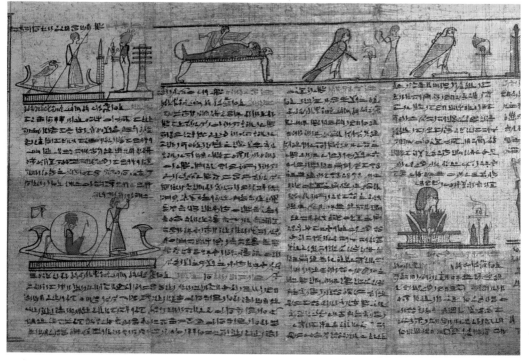

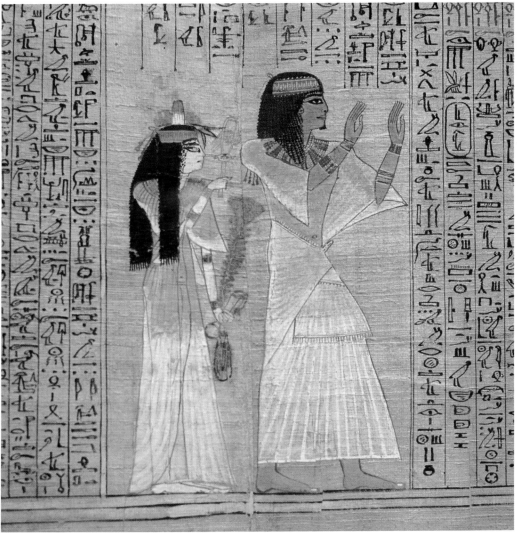

In 1250 BC this *Book of the Dead* from Thebes was made (extract) by the scribe Ani, which shows him and his wife praying to Osiris. The Egyptians thought the underworld (Duat) was similar to their land, with one river in the middle, and was to have been made of twelve regions following the twelve hours of the night. These regions were separated by gates, guarded by frightful creatures. For this reason the book of the dead is also known as the *Book of Gates*. Through the regions of the Duat and their terrible events, Egyptians made the trip to the underworld until the morning shone. *British Museum, London.*

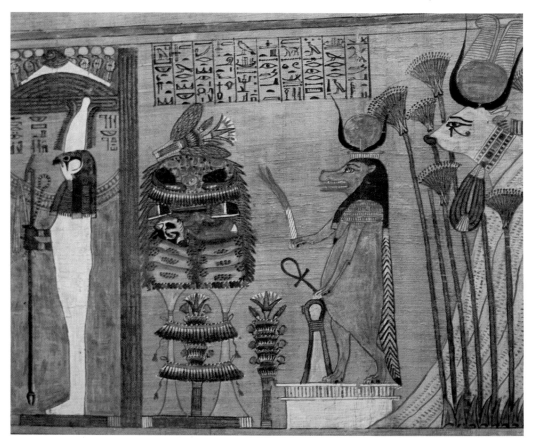

This papyrus of the dead was found in Thebes. It is supposed to represent Horus, with an Atef crown and in the form of Osiris. Behind him is a large flower or decorated "food offering," then Taweret as a pregnant "mixed being" (cross between a hippopotamus and a lion), and also Hathor as a cow in a lotus thicket. The papyrus was made around 1400 BC. *British Museum, London.*

good weather and hot days in Egypt should not obscure the fact that the nights were very cold. Spores of tuberculosis have been found on many mummies, and the singer Har-Mose must have already died of bronchopneumonia (bronchitis leads to the related infiltration of the lung tissue) before the infarct could announce itself. Leca wrote, "His right lung when placed in a tub with water sank instead of floated, a significant finding for physicians."

Women's diseases were numerous, lepra and pest appeared regularly, Ramses V had a severe hernia which infiltrated the scrotum, pushed it down, and doubled the size. Spinal cord arthroses were at the time as frequent as today, as were ligament injuries which we attribute today to our lengthy automobile driving habits. Wounds and fractures were also the order of the day.

Mummies as medications

One of the most perverse chapters of the history of medicine shall be discussed here at the end of this chapter: mummy fever in Europe. After the conquest of the pharaonic kingdom by the Romans, the priesthood no longer supervised the necropolis. Many thousands of tombs were totally plundered. With the arrival of Christianity, priests and monks destroyed the "pagan" tombs, emptied the vaults, and used the sarcophagi and mummies as fire material. During the Middle Ages and in the Renaissance, a "mummy fever" started. Mummies were offered as medicine against paralysis, weak heart, cough, epilepsy, bone fractures, and bruises. Mummy skin, mummy paste, and mummy powder were sold as a cure for liver and spleen disease, nausea, migraine and abscesses, and very nearly everything. This was started mainly by a Jewish physician by the name of El-Magar, who practiced in Alexandria around AD 1300 and who prescribed a "mummy" for any disease of his patients.

The "medicine" was provided either in the form of a part of a corpse or as an oily paste, which often had nothing to do with a mummy but instead was Jewish bitumen or asphalt called "tomb balsam." In the literature, four types of mummy remedies are described: "Arab mummies: a liquid of aloe, myrrh, and tomb balsam as found in tombs. From Egyptian mummies: a liquid that drips from corpses of small people that had been treated with asphalt—these mummies had been found in part completely intact. Artificial pissasphalt: a mixture of tar and bitumen, that was sold as the 'true mummy.' And, finally from the corpses buried in the sand and dried by the sun." The last two were cheaper since they did not require solution in resin or oil.

Savary de Bruslon recommended at the beginning of the seventeenth century, "the best mummies are those that do not shine, are almost black, smell good, and even on burning do not smell of tar."

Instructions for use are also found with the Arab alchemists, but let us restrict ourselves to our own pharmacist. In Becher's *Parnassus Medicalis Illustratus* of 1663 is the following recipe: "The mummy solves curdled blood / from spleen infection and cough it is good / swelling and wind of the belly / delayed women's time / you open two fifths / be prepared to pulverize." He indicates no difference between "true mummy meat" (ie, mummies from the desert of Egypt) and mummies made artificially out of fresh human meat. He maintained the latter was of greater usefulness than those coming from the desert. He also gave the recipe of how artificial mummies should be made: "One takes a boy, healthy / and wherever it can be / red-haired / a person killed by a rope / is placed one day in the sun / and one night in the rays of the moon." Then he can be dissolved. His flesh is cleaned and cut in long slices. These are treated with the addition of myrrh and aloe and digested with wine and alcohol (no heat) for eight to ten days. Finally, the individual parts are dried. Becher then concludes his description of the preparation, "It is totally without bad odor, lovely, and does not run on wet places."

One ordered mummies in ointments, balsams, tinctures, and extracts; sometimes as many as five types of mummies were supposed to have been used. Also, complete persons were used for medicinal purposes "with skin, meat, legs, everything." One crushed the whole individual to pulp "in a large mortar or several smaller ones" and made "aqua divina." From this, one gave to the sick a drachma with three to nine drops of his own blood added. Then relief should quickly result. One also made a drink for epilepsy by mixing stomach content and earth (told by George Buschan, "About medical magic and cures in the life of the people," Berlin, 1941).

It was a major spectacle to observe where the mummy shipments were sent. The mummies were transported in caravans on mules and camels to Cairo and Alexandria where they were placed on Portuguese and Venetian ships and sent to France. The center for mummy commerce was apparently Lyon, from where the shipment of mummies to pharmacies all over the land was organized. Resale took place at very high prices.

Mummies were not to "rest in peace" for centuries, because it was very fashionable in horror- and ghost-happy England to be invited to a "mummy dinner." The height of the meal and of the evening was the unwrapping of a real mummy. In Germany, at the same time, it was possible to be part owner of a "real Egyptian mummy" for twenty Reichsmarks. And the fate of mummies in the United States was not enviable. At the end of the nineteenth century, the merchant August Stanwood, who had paper factories in Maine, had the idea of making paper out of cloth rags. He bought mummies from Arabs who had experience in this commerce, unwrapped them, and started his business with corpse bandages and cloth. Unfortunately, the resin acted on the cloth such that the paper coming from the machines was brown, not white. Stanwood could not find any method to make the paper white, so this smart man sold his paper as wrapping paper. Thus, the American housewife brought her food home in the "cloth of the mummies." What happened to the mummies we do not know. The ancient Egyptians only wanted to remain in their vaults and tombs forever and always to sail in peace on Re's sun barge!

Epilogue

Man is scared of time—
Time is scared of the pyramids.
(Egyptian proverb)

After a late lunch, from the terrace of my hotel I was able to observe the mountains behind the Nile and the harsh landscape of the West where so many tombs of pharaohs were hewed into the stone. As at many other times, the first glance of the view fascinated me anew. Under an amethyst-blue sky, the mountains shone in mauve; filled with riddles, soon they would look as though they were painted in purple when the sun abruptly sank into the underworld. The day in the Valley of the Kings was, as always, glowing. Rock, rubble, and sand of the desert do not offer shade. In the tombs it is hot and sticky. The sweat of the visitors damages the wall paintings. Thus, even if the visitors do not actually touch the artifacts to discover whether they are real or not, damage is done. The tomb cities need "vacations" from the tourists. Hence, half are always closed due to restoration or atmospheric problems.

These problems did not exist when the city of Thebes, the grandiose city of the dead, was created in view of the world. Vainly one searches for a trace of those who became similar to the gods under the mountain points of the West in an imposing neighborhood for the dead.

The sacred city no longer exists with its ram's heads, with its alleys and suburbs in which the embalmers and the workers for the gigantic necropolis lived and dealt with mummies, the city with colossal statues, columns, masts and pillars, with the Ramesseum, and with the many small gardens in which the souls rested when they came out from the well of the tombs into the light of the world. Only the view remains where the yellow sand becomes the green of the meadows and where there is a stream and stony waterfalls.

When did they disappear—those sacred barges and their garrison and the 180 thousand men of Thebes who only worked for Amun (as sculptors, stone workers, papyrus pressers, or caretakers of fowl, in the smelting ovens and the writing halls, at the sacred sea, in the forbidden area or the area of the sick)? Thebes, the city that once swallowed Luxor, which stretched all the way to the horizon on one side and on the other to Karnak, the oasis that was transformed into stone, does not exist any more. Today we sit in the glowing evening light. Delicate hoopoe make holes in the horse apples that are lying on the sidewalk. The tourists ride in one-horse vehicles into Karnak, which was called Ipet-isut, the "outer side of the shadow," the ideologically and economically most important temple untertaking in all of Egypt. But testimonials in ruins do not die, and a language can be found again. Like Champollion, who at his arrival in Upper Egypt enthusiastically claimed, "Thebes is the biggest word that exists in any language." And Karnak opens the majesty of the pharaohs' kingdom. It is the largest that humankind has thought of and created. No other people of ancient times knew the art of architecture at such a high level and with such high standards.

The pharaohs were not able to completely conquer death. From their cities of death, from Biban el-Muluk, they might have watched the building of Karnak, its constant enlargement and beautification, and finally its destruction by boots of foreign soldiers.

For the pharaoh, Karnak was more than a temple-city. Here he found his legitimacy, here he came to find comfort and hope after strikes of misfortune. Here he brought his victories to Amun as homage, and here he found new energy. After all, he was only a leaf from the tree whose majestic roots were anchored in the soil of Thebes, and whose stories we still hear today.

At the end of the dynasties, the decay and disintegration of the Egyptian realm could not be stopped. Incense was still burned, homage and embalming were brought to the gods, the Nile flowed over and then regressed. However, the knowledge, art, and science in all forms disappeared. Wars were fought with mercenaries; it was as if the country wanted to fall into a perpetual sleep. Egypt became drunk with lethargy.

As Alexander the Great

and later the Romans marched in, medical literature did not suddenly stop. There was a continuation of the writing of medical recipes—in the Coptic language of the Egyptian Christians. Naturally, this medicine was already influenced by the Greeks, since everything the Greeks did rose from Egypt. Even Hippocrates admitted how much he relied on the knowledge of ancient Egyptian physicians.

Even if Egyptian medicine depended on Arabic medicine, it retained a certain Egyptian tradition with words and concepts which otherwise probably would have been lost. In particular one must thank the cloisters for carefully treating the old texts. For example, many medical recipes were found in the cloister Deir el-Abjad. In 1921 a manuscript of the ninth (or tenth) century AD was published that had been found in Meshaikh by M. E. Bouriant—a handwritten manuscript on eye diseases that is very similar to that of old Egyptian papyri. At the time this manuscript from Meshaikh was written, Greek medicine had already passed its zenith, and Arab medicine was heading toward new and fruitful horizons.

For 2,500 years, the Nile flowed after the physician Imhotep had built the first pyramid in Saqqara for his pharaoh, Djoser. Lotus and papyrus were faded, mighty Memphis was forgotten. In AD 969, far from Memphis in the fields of Dschaubar Misr al-Kahira, today's Cairo was built. Shiny mosques were built to the honor and fame of Allah, "the kindest, the only God who created the World."

While humankind paid homage to Allah, the desert kindly covered the cities of Amun and his followers. Only the highest constructions remained as the wonders of the world, visible at all times, disturbingly secretive.

The culture, however, in those distant days from the first dynasty on, did suddenly shine on Europe and Africa and was not in any way dead. The culture inspired art, handiwork, literature, and medicine, even until today.

Ever since Champollion unlocked the mystery of hieroglyphics, and the spades of archaeologists discovered marvelous secrets, we have sat in admiration of the largest culture of our creation.

Glossary

We tried as much as possible in this book to exclude technical terms, or else we tried to explain them in the text. Other words are explained in the following list. In addition there are more details about official positions, titles, or priest matters for the interested reader.

Abydos Main cult of Osiris, allegedly with his tomb. City of the tombs of kings of the First and Second Dynasties.

alabaster After the Egyptian city Alabastron. Transparent, white, yellow, red, or gray mineral that was used in Egyptian and Babylonian times for vases and reliefs.

Amaunet Founding goddess, the female counterpart of Amun and in Ptolemy's time "North wind."

Amenti Kingdom of the dead.

Amun Main deity of Thebes. For 2,000 years was considered the only god of creation.

ankham Life. A flower garland that gave the dead the divine life force.

ankh sign A hieroglyphic key on tombs or coffins. Symbol of life and vigor. Christian "handle cross."

Anubis Jackal-headed necropolis god "responsible" for mummification.

apis The sacred steer with the sun disk between its horns. Associated with Ptah.

Ba Force in man outlasting death; often not quite correctly translated as soul. The Ba of the dead moved around freely in the other world and is represented by the figure of a bird.

Bastet Lion-headed war goddess closely associated with Nut and Sakhmet.

Bes Dwarf with mask, god of the family and protector of pregnant women.

cartouche Oval with cross-beams in which the name of the king was written, starting from the Fourth Dynasty onwards. The kings had two cartouche names; one referred to the Throne name, the other the name at birth.

cataract Hard stony region in the bed of a river that results in rapids. Six in number between Aswan and Kartoum. Hazardous to navigation, the second could only be navigated during a flood. At different times also a land boundary.

Chepre God of creation in the form of a beetle.

Champollion Jean-Francois. Solved the riddle of the hieroglyphs in 1822.

demotic Continuation of the development of hieratic folk writing and everyday writing in the late time.

district Administrative unit with the name "sepat." These units had a major role when the kingdom was administered strongly, for example during the Middle Kingdom. Regional princes and not very important people were the highest officers, hereditary from the Twelfth Dynasty.

Duat The underworld that disappears in the sun in order to traverse it.

Geb Belonged to the "nine ones of Heliopolis"; god personality of the Earth and husband of the sky goddess Nut. Directed the first scribes of the dead in the underworld.

Harakhty "Horus of the horizon," is represented as a human with a falcon head.

Harpokrates Always represented as a naked child, with a finger in his mouth and children's locks of hair. Son of Isis and Osiris.

Hathor With sun disk and cow horns, goddess of women, also goddess of heaven, tree goddess (Memphis), and necropolis goddess.

Heliopolis Important place of religion and closely associated with the sun cult. In Egyptian: "Junu"; in Bible: "On."

Heracleopolis   Scene of the fight between Seth and Horus.

hieratic   Customary writing for papyri and ostraka. Simpler to write than hieroglyphs.

hieroglyphs   Greek "sacred notch"; identifiable picture language, usually only on monuments.

Horus   Represented as falcon headed and often with the double crown of Upper and Lower Egypt. God of heaven and one of the group of nine of Heliopolis. Son of Isis and Osiris.

Imhotep   Physician, sculptor, and architect for Pharaoh Djoser of the first pyramid of the world in Saqqara; "raised" to god status.

Isis   Sister and wife of Osiris (dying sun) and mother of Horus (newborn sun). Grants protection to the dead.

Jaru   Land of the other side of blest where the dead continue to live, plough, eat, drink, and love.

Ka   Life vigor that accompanies people like a "double." Guarantees eternal life.

Ker-heb priests   Reading priests in the dead cult of embalmer during mummification of the corpse.

Khnum   Ram-headed god of creation, sometimes represented in pictures of people at the potter's wheel.

Maat   Goddess with ostrich feather. Personification of truth. At the death tribunal the heart of the deceased was weighed in the Maat balance.

mastaba   Arabic for "bank." Used for the name of freestanding stepped graves in the Old Kingdom.

Min   God of fertility. Represented with a cap with two feathers, scourge, and erect penis. Protector of the east desert.

necropolis   Greek for cemetery. City of the dead with extended surface for burial, usable for a prolonged time.

Neith   Goddess of war with arrow, arch, and shield. Together with Isis, Nephthys, and Selket the guards at the litter of Osiris.

Nephthys   Sister of Isis, with whom she always appears.

Nine, the   Group of nine gods in several cultures. The great group of nine of Heliopolis was Re-Atum, Shu, Tefnut, Geb, Nut, Osiris, Isis, Sweth, and Nephthys.

Nun   Personification of original water from which Earth was created.

Nut   Goddess of heaven and mother of Re, the sun god.

obelisk   Monument with right angles and diminishing size as it rises upwards to stone arrow. Probably a sun symbol; appears before graves in pairs; single ones are objects. Obelisks are of one piece and now are in New York, Paris, and Munich.

Osiris Mummy figure with curved staff, scourge, and a white crown over ram horns. God of vegetation, rhythm, and the underworld. Divided into pieces and put together again by Isis.

ostrakon Greek for potter's wheel. Clay wheel that was used for making round pads for scribes and designers; 20,000 were found, of which the best were of the Nineteenth and Twentieth Dynasties.

papyrus Base for writing, made by pressing papyrus stalks together.

pharaoh From Egyptian Per'o ("great house"). Title of the Egyptian king.

pylon Monumental entrance wall of temples, usually two massive towers with arches. Extended temples usually have several pylons.

Re (Ra) Sun god, who travels in the sun barge over the heaven accompanied by Thoth and his daughter, Maat. The dead also traveled in the barge of Re.

Sakhmet Lion-headed goddess associated with Nut and Bastet.

Sekhem Powerful being. "Things

that Sekhem knows" means they are "similar to the gods."

sempriest High priest, who at the ritual of the opening of the mouth had the role of the god Horus and wore a panther skin.

Seth God of chaos, the desert, the storm, and war. Unidentified animal brother of Osiris.

Shu Master of the air, master of the four winds.

Sobek Crocodile god who from the Middle Kingdom on was deemed as powerful as Horus.

Sokaris As god of the necropolis was stationed at the entrance of the underworld. God of the dead, who later equaled Osiris. Festive dead celebrations were held using a "Sokaris-barge."

Sothis The star, Sirius, which appeared in the sky in early summer and indicated the beginning of the flood of the Nile.

Taweret The pregnant hippopotamus goddess with female breasts. Protector goddess of pregnant women.

Tefnut Female representation of Shu.

Thoth God of the moon and science, knowledge, and date determination. Represented with ibis head or as a baboon, and in the company of Re during the day.

uraeus   The golden serpents used on the foreheads of kings. Sacred animals that represented the eye of the sun.

uschebti   Small figures which were given to mummies in the tombs. Par-tial representations of the deceased with as many as 365 in a tomb—one figure for each day, in case the pharaoh needed workers in the underworld.

uzat (or udjat) eye   Favorite amulet placed in the tomb. Symbol of cyclical renewal of life, to protect the carrier from the unexpected.

References

Ankylostomiasis and Bilharziasis in Egypt. Cairo, Egypt: Government Press; 1972.

Bauer W, Dümotz I, Golowin S. *Lexikon der Symbole.* Munich, Germany: Heyne; 1987.

Bauer H. *5000 Jahre Medizinische Entdeckungen und Entdecker.* Leipzig, Germany: Brockhaus Verlag; 1954.

Baumann H. *Die Welt der Pharaonen. Entdecker am Nil.* Gütersloh, Germany: Mohn; 1959.

Bekker J. Essay to Diodor I,/8. Leipzig, Germany: Teubner, 1853.

Bissing FWV. *Altägyptische Lebensweisheit.* Zürich, Switzerland: Artemis-Verlag; 1955.

The Book of the Dead. Commentaries by Evelyn Rossiter. British Museum. London, England: Regent; Paris, France: Seghers; 1978.

Brandenburg D. *Medizinisches bei Herodot.* Berlin, Germany: Hessling-Verlag; 1976.

Breasted JH. *Journal of Egyptian Archaeology.* London, 1949.

Brunner-Traut E. *Die alten Ägypter—Verborgenes Leben und Pharaonen.* Stuttgart, Germany: Verlag W. Kohlhammer; 1974.

Buschan G. *About Medical Magic and Cures in the Life of the People.* Berlin, Germany: Obis; 1941.

Capart J. *L'Art Egyptien. Études et Histoire.* Brussel: L'Institut Français d'Archéologie; 1924.

Carter H. *The Tomb of Tut-ankh-Amen.* London, England: Arena; license Brockhaus, Wiesbaden, Germany; 1933.

Cattrell L. *Das Volk der Pharaonen.* Stuttgart, Germany: Diana Verlag; 1965.

Champdor A. *Das Ägyptische Totenbuch.* Munich, Germany: Manfred Lurker, Verlag Droemer-Knaur; 1977.

David AR. *Ancient Egypt.* Oxford, England: Phaidon; 1988.

David AR. *The Pyramid Builders of Ancient Egypt: A Modern Investigation of Pharaoh's Workforce.* London, England: Aris & Phillips; 1986.

De Buck A. *Die godsdienstige opvattning van den slaap inzonderheid in het oude Egypte.* Leiden, The Netherlands: Brill; 1939.

de Denon DV. *Mit Napoleon in Ägypten 1798–1799.* Hrsg Helmut Arndt. Munich/Zürich: Knaur, and Tübingen: Erdmann; 1982.

Diepgen P. *Geschichte der Medizin. Die historische Entwicklung der Heilkunde und des ärztlichen Lebens. Band I: Von den Anfängen bis zum 18. Jahrhundert.* Berlin, Germany: Verlag Gruyter; 1949.

Ebers G. *Papyrus Ebers. Das hermetische Buch über die Arzneimittel der Alten Ägypterin hieratischer Schrift. Band I und II.* Leipzig, Germany: Verlag Engelmann; 1879.

Ebers G. *Eine ägyptische Königstochter.* 3 Bände. Stuttgart/Leipzig, Germany: Hallberger; 1879.

el Dawakhly Z, Ghalioungui P. *Health and Healing in Ancient Egypt.* Cairo, Egypt: Dar Al-Maaref; 1965.

Eriksson M, Sjolund B. *Transkutane Nervenstimulierung zur Schmerzlinderung.* Heidelberg, Germany: Fischer; 1979.

Erman A. *Literatur der Ägypter.* Leipzig, Germany: Verlag de Gruyter; 1923.

Eydt M. *Kampf um die Cheops-Pyramide—Geschichten aus dem Leben eines Ingenieurs.* Zwei Bände der Carl Winter's Universitätsbuchhandlung Heidelberg. (Die letzte Recherche des Autors nach der Herkunft der Bücher weist einen handschriftlichen "Gotthelf Wülber" als Besitzer aus. Das 840-Seiten-Werk lag 1979 zum Verkauf im Kairoer Khan-el-Khalili-Basar und wurde—vielleicht etwa um die Jahrhundertwende—abgestempelt von der "Buchhandlung Crone & Martinot, Hamburg—St. Pauli, neben der Post.")

Flaubert G. *Notes inédits … Voyage d'Egypte 1849–51.* Hrsg Dr G. A. Narciss, nach der Ausgabe von 1920. Frankfurt/Stuttgart, Germany: Fischer/Bertelsmann; 1963, 1978.

Gardiner AH. *Egyptian Grammar.* 3rd ed. Oxford, England: Oxford University Press; 1957.

Grapow H. *Grundriss der Medizin der alten Ägypter.* Berlin, Germany: Akademie-Verlag; 1954.

Grapow H. *Über die anatomischen Kenntnisse der altägyptischen Ärzte.* Beitrag in Heft 26 von "Morgenland—Darstellungen aus Geschichte und Kultur des Ostens." Leipzig, Germany: Hinrichs; 1935.

Harris JE. *X-raying the Pharaohs.* Chicago: University of Chicago Press; 1973.

Harris JE. *An X-ray Atlas of the Royal Mummies.* Chicago: University of Chicago Press; 1980.

Hatem A-K. *Life in Ancient Egypt.* Cairo, Egypt: Al Ahram; 1982.

Hermann A. *Ägyptische Liebesdichtung.* Wiesbaden, Germany: Verlag Otto Harrassowitz; 1959.

Herodot. *Historien II.* Munich, Germany: Heimeran; 1977.

Irmscher J. *Lexikon der Antike.* Munich, Germany: Heyne; 1987.

Jacq C. *Akhenaton et Nefertiti.* Paris, France: Laffont; 1976.

Kayer H. *100 Tore hatte Theben. Historische Stätten am Nil.* Hannover, Germany: Fackelträger-Verlag; 1965.

Kluge M. *Weisheit der alten Ägypter.* Munich, Germany: Heyne; 1980.

Kluzinger CB. *Pictures Out of Upper Egypt.* Cairo, Egypt: Kluzinger; 1877.

Kraemer H (Hrsg). *Weltall und Menschheit. Geschichte der Erforschung der Natur und der Verwertung der Naturkräfte im Dienste der Völker. Band III: Prof Karl Weule; Band IV: Dr Albert Neuburger.* Bonn/Berlin/Leipzig/Wien, Germany: Dt. Verlagshaus.

Konzelmann G. *Der Nil.* Hamburg, Germany: Hoffmann und Campe; 1982.

Leca A-P. *Die Mumien.* Berlin, Germany: Ullstein; 1984.

Lefebvre G. *Tableau des Parties du Corps Humain Mentionnées par les Egyptiens.* Supp 17 in "Annales du Service des Antiquités de l'Egypte. Cairo, Egypt: Sasae; 1952.

Lichtenthaler C. *Geschichte der Medizin. Die Reihenfolge ihrer Epochenbilder und die treibenden Kräfte. Band 1.* Köln/Lövenich, Germany: Deutscher Ärzteverlag; 1974.

Magnus H. *Die Augenheilkunde der Alten.* Breslau, Germany: J.U. Kern; 1901.

Maspero G. *Les Inscriptions des Pyramides de Saqquarah.* Paris, France: Etudes de Mythologie et de Archéologie Egyptiennes, Bd. I; 1893.

Mendelssohn K. *The Riddle of the Pyramids.* London, England: Thames & Hudson; 1974.

Montet P. *So lebten die Ägypter vor 3000 Jahren.* Stuttgart, Germany: Deutsche Verlagsanstalt; 1960.

Montlauer P. *Imhotep.* Reinbek, Germany: Rowohlt-Verlag; 1988.

Morenz S. *Die Begegnung Europas mit Ägypten.* Mit einem Beitrag von Martin Kaiser über Herodots Begegnung mit Ägypten. Zürich/Stuttgart, Germany: Artemis Verlag; 1969.

Morenz S. *Religion und Geschichte der alten Ägypter.* Köln/Wien, Germany: Verlag Bohlau; 1975.

Paullini T. *Neuvermehrte heilsame Dreckapotheke.* Frankfurt/Main, Germany: Paullini.

Petrie WMF. *The Royal Tombs of the Earliest Dynasties. London, England: Egyptian Archeology; 1901.*

Ranke H. Medizin und Chirurgie im alten Ägypten. Heidelberg, Germany: Heidelberger Vorträge, Universität Heidelberg; 1948.

Ramadura E. *Das alte ägyptische Traumbuch.* Darmstadt, Germany: Bergewald-Verlag; 1988.

Ruffer MA. *Studies in the Paleopathology of Egypt.* Chicago, Ill: Roy L. Moodie; 1921.

Sameh WWDS. *Alltag im alten Ägypten.* Munich, Germany: Callwey; 1963.

Saunderon S. *Les Songes et leur interpretation dans L'Egypte ancienne.* Paris, France: Hazan; 1959.

Schenkel W. *Grundformen mittelägyptischer Sätze anhand der Sinuhe-Erzählung.* Berlin, Germany: Hessling-Verlag; 1965.

Schipperges H. *Moderne Medizin im Spiegel der Geschichte.* Stuttgart, Germany: Deutscher Taschenbuch-Verlag. Band 4044, wissenschaftliche Reihe; 1970.

Schipperges H. *Lebendige Heilkunde von großen Ärzten und Philosophen aus drei Jahrtausenden.* Freiburg, Germany: Olten; 1962.

Schüssler K. *Märchen und Erzählungen der alten Ägypter.* Lübbe: Bergisch Gladbach; 1980.

Sethe K. *Origin of the Eighteenth Dynasty.* Leipzig, Germany: Verlag Engelmann; 1914.

Sigerist HE. *Anfänge der Medizin. Von der primitiven und archaischen Medizin bis zum goldenen Zeitalter.* Zürich, Switzerland: Europa Verlag; 1963.

Sigerist HE. *Große Ärzte. Eine Geschichte der Heilkunde in Lebensbildern.* Munich, Germany: J.F. Lehmann; 1965.

Smith GE. *A Contribution to the Study of Mummification in Egypt.* Vol 5. Cairo, Egypt: Memoires de l'Institut Egyptien; 1906.

Spiegel J. *Das Werden der altägyptischen Hochkultur. Ägyptische Geistesgeschichte im 3. Jahrtausend n. Chr.* Heidelberg, Germany: Kerle; 1953.

Thorwald J. *Macht und Geheimnis der frühen Ärzte.* Munich, Germany/Zürich, Switzerland: Knaur/Taschenbuch 138; 1967.

Tulhoff A. *Thutmosis III.* Munich, Germany: Callwey; 1984.

Vandenberg P. *Ramses der Große.* Bern/Munich: Scherz; Lübbe: Gladbach; 1980.

References

von Däniken E. *Die Augen der Sphinx*. Munich, Germany: Bertelsmann; 1989.

von Deines H. *Übersetzung der medizinischen Texte*. Berlin, Germany: Akademischer Verlag; 1958.

Waltari M. *Sinuhe der Ägypter*. Bern, Switzerland: Lindenverlag; 1948.

Westendorf W. *Lexikon der Ägyptologie*. Wiesbaden, Germany: Verlag Otto Harrassowitz; Bd I–Bd VI, 1975–1986.

Zabkar LV. *A Study of the Ba Concept*. Chicago: University of Chicago Press; 1968.

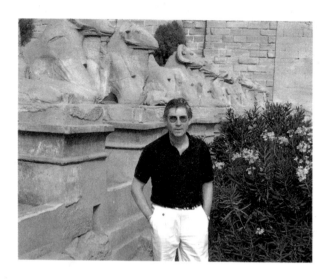

About the Author

Cornelius Stetter is a professional journalist. For the past 20 years, he has traveled around the world as a medical author as well as a magazine reporter. His reports have brought him in contact with Presidents Anwar el-Sadat and Hosni Mubarak in Egypt. He was present when the first legendary mummy hall in Cairo was closed, which gave him the idea for this book. In the following years, Stetter, who was born in Munich, investigated all the scenes of Mediterranean medical history, as well as local universities and libraries. This compendium, which describes people and physicians from 4,500 years ago, was supported by Egyptian ministries and countless scientists.